About the Author

SHREVE STOCKTON is a professional photographer whose work has been published in numerous magazines and displayed in galleries from Los Angeles to New York. Diagnosed with celiac disease early in 2003, Stockton has devoted herself to learning everything she can about managing and cooking for gluten intolerance. She lives in San Francisco.

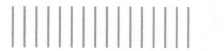

EATING

GLUTEN FREE

EATING

GLUTEN FREE

Delicious Recipes and Essential Advice
for Living Well without Wheat and
Other Problematic Grains

SHREVE STOCKTON

FOREWORD BY Danna Korn

MARLOWE & COMPANY
NEW YORK

EATING GLUTEN FREE: *Delicious Recipes and Essential Advice for Living Well without Wheat and Other Problematic Grains*

Copyright © 2005 Shreve Stockton
Foreword copyright © 2005 Danna Korn

Published by
Marlowe & Company
An Imprint of Avalon Publishing Group Incorporated
245 West 17th Street • 11th floor
New York, NY 10011

AVALON
publishing group incorporated

Library of Congress Control Number: 2004116087

ISBN 1-56924-393-X

9 8 7 6 5 4 3 2

Designed by Pauline Neuwirth, Neuwirth and Associates, Inc.

Printed in Canada
Distributed by Publishers Group West

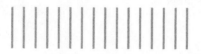

Contents

Foreword by Danna Korn   ix

PART ONE: **The Handbook**   1

   Introduction   3
1 From Misery to Gluten Free   5
2 No Grain, No Pain: Gluten Intolerance Demystified   8
3 A Healthy Choice for Every Body   16
4 Don't Move! You Might Be Near Gluten   19
5 Making the Transition   27
6 Kitchen Essentials   36
7 Excursions and Adventures   41

PART TWO: **The Recipes**   45

   Breakfast and Brunch   47
   Smoothies   55
   Breads   77
   Soups   93
   Salads and Sides   111
   Entrées   135

Sweets   159
Marinades and Dressings   173

  Resources   183
  For Further Reading   185
  Acknowledgments   187
  Index   189

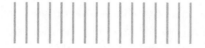

Foreword

by Danna Korn

The wheat-free/gluten-free diet is one of the fastest-growing nutritional trends in America. And it's no wonder! Millions of people are discovering that the wheat-free/gluten-free diet is the key to better health. After all, wheat really isn't good for anyone.

Admittedly, the wheat-free/gluten-free diet can be daunting, especially at first. But with an open mind, a shift in perspective, accurate information, and a touch of inspiration, most people discover that it's easier than they imagined it would be.

The most important element of learning to live (and love) the gluten-free lifestyle is attitude. You can curse the diet because it has its limitations; or you can be thankful that those limitations allow you to enjoy improved health and vitality. It's important to remember to focus on the reasons this diet is a *good* thing in your life. One of the best ways to do that is to arm yourself with accurate information and helpful resources.

When I embarked upon this lifestyle in 1991, there were few resources available. There was no Internet. There were no books. The support groups I found were wonderful, but they were for adults—and at that time, my needs were focused on raising my celiac son, still just a toddler. The gluten-free products that were available then were—ahem—a little less than savory, and little more than inedible, *if* one could afford them. And asking for help from manufacturers or store staff was an exercise in futility.

Today, the situation is dramatically improved. There are excellent Web sites and books, support groups, awareness campaigns, and new labeling laws. The quality and accessibility of gluten-free products has gone up, while prices have come down. But most importantly, there has been a shift from thinking of this diet as a curse to realizing that it's a cure. Optimism is pervasive, and it's key for dealing with this lifestyle in a productive, healthy manner. The ultimate reward—improved health and vitality—is the incentive that will keep you on track.

Once I got a handle on how to deal with the diet and the unique challenges it presented, it became clear that my future would be blessed with the privilege of reaching out and helping others.

Author Shreve Stockton has obviously done the same thing with *Eating Gluten Free*. A unique blend of information and recipes, including helpful cooking and preparation hints, *Eating Gluten Free* is more than just a cookbook . . . more than a handbook . . . it's an outstanding addition to the library of anyone on a wheat-free/gluten-free diet.

DANNA KORN is the author of *Wheat-Free, Worry-Free: The Art of Happy, Healthy, Gluten-Free Living* and *Kids with Celiac Disease: A Family Guide to Raising Happy, Healthy, Gluten-Free Children* and the founder of R.O.C.K. (Raising Our Celiac Kids). Visit www.gluten-freedom.net and www.celiackids.com for more information.

ONE

The Handbook

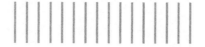

Introduction

As a rule, cookbooks are created by people who love to cook. Welcome to the exception. I have always had a steadfast aversion to all things kitchen; for 10 years, I used my oven for storage and didn't even own any plates. Everything changed once I realized I was gluten intolerant. I was forced to bake if I wanted any bread or cookies or pancakes, and cook in order to dine without worry.

After being ill for months, I was thrilled to feel *alive* again and to achieve this renewed health by simply changing what I ate. However, my happiness slowly turned to panic once I understood what the future involved. The convenience of ordering out was no longer an option, restaurants were filled with potential dangers, and the meager array of expensive gluten-free products available in grocery stores left much to be desired. This lead to the most terrifying realization of all: I would have to cook. Though confusion and anxiety infused my foray into cooking, though many of my early attempts yielded nothing but inedible hockey pucks, though tears of anger seasoned many a dish, I eventually realized that cooking was just an opportunity to be creative. Since then I have learned much and eaten well.

Health is about how you feel and how you function—it's about working *with* your body to live as vibrant and fulfilling a life as possible. There is no denying how traumatizing it is to realize that you may never again allow wheat or gluten to pass your lips. Yet the transformation that occurs when you make that commitment is remarkable. This book is here to make that transition easier: to reinforce the choices you will need to make in order to stay well, to show that *anything* new can be exciting and inspiring, and, above all, to demonstrate that this condition, and the lifestyle shift it demands, can bring about the most intense joy, health, and vivacity you have ever experienced.

I

FROM MISERY TO
GLUTEN FREE

My own intolerance to gluten caused the most agonizing six months I've ever endured. Though the experience was incredibly difficult to overcome, it had the most amazing effect on my life, and through it, I have gained enormous insight. Addressing my gluten intolerance led to profound and lasting changes, both physically and deep within my psyche, which immediately began taking place once I removed gluten from my diet.

Now that I understand things, I can pinpoint when and why my gluten intolerance began. It started spontaneously, triggered by stress. I was moving across the country, leaving a city I was madly in love with for a city I had dreamt about my entire life. I was relocating my business, reuniting with my dearest friend, becoming a "third parent" to my godson, and using all my savings to start this venture. It was a huge risk, and one I knew was worthwhile.

Right before I left, I began having sharp pains in my abdomen, so severe they would wake me from my sleep. Fearing appendicitis, I went to the emergency room and was told it was a muscle strain. The pain persisted and I ignored it long enough to finalize my move, pack a moving van in minus-10-degree weather, and arrive in my new city, a spinning top of shock, excitement, and pain.

I knew something was very wrong inside of me. The sharp stabbing pains alternated with a constant dull ache that became a backdrop to my life. At times, it was so bad that I couldn't walk or stand upright. I lived with this until I was settled enough in my new life to find a gastroenterologist. After hearing my symptoms and doing a brief physical, the doctor told me that what I was experiencing was a by-product of stress, and if I did not chill out, I should start taking Xanax. He thought I might have an ulcer and ordered blood tests and a barium X-ray to confirm this.

I refused the drugs, all tests for the ulcer came back negative, and my gastroenterologist said there was nothing else to do.

Meanwhile, it felt like I was sinking into hell. The pain, confusion, and depression that plagued me in the months before I learned I was gluten intolerant were unparalleled. While my physical distress was significant, the neurological effects were the most severe: unyielding months of days unbroken by joy, the sludge of exhaustion, the overall despondency that kept me from my life, and an unbearable confusion when my attempts to overcome my given state afforded no change. I tried everything to combat my depression and to override the fatigue. Knowing that exercise alleviates listlessness and depression, I would force myself to go running, do yoga, bicycle across town. However, because of the undiagnosed gluten intolerance, my body was not getting the adequate nutrition to handle even sedentary days. I began to experience heavier and heavier fatigue, and an absolutely debilitating depression. The mere act of existing became a trial of endurance. I slept a ridiculous amount, at least nine hours a night plus a three-hour nap every day. My level of fatigue reached a point where I had to lie on the bathroom floor while brushing my teeth. I felt like I was in some sort of living coma. I would shut myself in my office and try to work, but work was excruciating because I could hardly concentrate. I would have to read something over and over in order to finally comprehend it. I had spent my life creating—quick to think, quick to act—and now even the simplest of tasks were daunting. I was so frustrated with myself. I thought I was having a spiritual crisis; it never occurred to me that it was a physical one. Meanwhile, my savings were dwindling, and I had no income because I no longer had the strength or mental capacity to work.

In a desperate attempt to make myself better, I decided to try a cleansing fast, a jump start for my aching soul. I researched fasting and found one that sounded safe and intelligent, consisting of nothing but water, fresh lemon juice, maple syrup, and cayenne pepper. I fully expected to feel even worse while on this fast: no food, no nourishment. Instead, I felt amazing. It was truly incredible, and at the time I could not believe it. I woke up every morning happy. Smiling and energized. Excited and driven. I got more accomplished in that week than I had in the previous four months. The irony: It was while I was eating that I was receiving no nutrition. The fast gave me a hiatus from unknowingly destroying my body. However, I was more confused and devastated than ever once I went off the fast and started eating again. Instantly, the pain and depression returned.

After five months, at the end of my rope, I rented a truck and drove to Death Valley. I spent a week alone in the heat and the emptiness, praying for a shift, for an understanding, for a way to heal. And during that week in the desert, I felt wonderful, with loads of energy and a vitality I had forgotten existed. All I ate during that trip was fruit, nuts, and corn cakes, all of which happen to be gluten free. I was scared to go home, scared that my wonderful feeling of well-being would end—and it did. It ended with my first piece of toast.

Three weeks later I had a follow-up appointment with my gastroenterologist and told him of the periods of feeling healthy and wonderful, once while fasting, once while camping. I knew there had to be a key to the problem in there somewhere. I kept pressing him about it, and he then mentioned, as an afterthought, the possibility of gluten intolerance. I had the blood tests, which came back inconclusive. I was told it would take weeks to schedule the biopsy. Unable to wait any longer to end the misery I was in, I researched celiac disease extensively and then cut out all gluten from my diet as a test. Within a matter of days my suffering was completely gone, and has never returned.

Living without gluten has been a fascinating experience for me. The immediate and marked changes that occurred once I eliminated gluten were astounding, and initially eclipsed any negative feelings I had about being gluten intolerant. I was just thrilled to feel alive again.

However, giving up gluten has its own set of pains, and I have broken down in tears at the health food store many times. The overwhelming magnitude of what is required to stay healthy is intimidating and demands more than willpower. It involves a complete restructuring of your entire life. The psychological transformations that come along with making a commitment this immense are subtle and mysterious. You begin to develop an awareness of your body, and of your actions, and of the consequences of your actions. Initially, this awareness is focused on your diet and your health, but by strengthening your will and awareness in one particular area, the practice inevitably grows to encompass all other areas of your life.

2

NO GRAIN, NO PAIN: GLUTEN INTOLERANCE DEMYSTIFIED

The moment of your diagnosis may very likely have been the first time you heard of gluten intolerance or celiac disease. Most people don't know such a condition exists until they have to deal with it firsthand. Though estimates show that at least 1 in 133 people have celiac disease, and that 90 million people in the United States—nearly one-third of the population—have some form of gluten intolerance, the vast majority of these people are undiagnosed. The lack of recognition regarding this condition can make it very confusing for those who learn they are gluten intolerant. Knowledge is essential to feel safe, informed, and less overwhelmed. It is important to understand gluten intolerance in order to combat the confusion and isolation that can so easily envelop you, and also to prevent naive but harmful mistakes. Sharing this information with your family, friends, and significant others will help you through your transition and may also shed light on someone else's struggle. The rate of diagnosis for celiac disease and gluten intolerance increases each year as doctors and the general public become more informed about the symptoms and dangers of this disease.

▪ Who Is Affected by Gluten Intolerance? ▪

Anyone can develop gluten intolerance, at any time during one's life. It can be triggered by stress, surgery, or pregnancy, though there is a genetic link as well. The extended family of anyone who has been diagnosed with gluten intolerance should be aware of their own predisposition and should seek the appropriate testing, regardless if they show symptoms or not. Gluten intolerance can be detected in toddlers and diagnosed in seniors, though the majority of new cases are women of child-bearing age. Most people do not know they are gluten intolerant and struggle with physical pain, chronic fatigue, unyielding depression, migraines, or a host of other ills and have no idea why. Some people have no obvious symptoms or may consider their discomfort normal. In any case, gluten intolerance causes damage within the body that can have serious consequences if left unchecked.

▪ What Is Gluten Intolerance? ▪

For those who are gluten intolerant, wheat, rye, barley, and oats are toxic. Gluten is the protein found in wheat, rye, and barley. While oats do not contain gluten, they are not considered gluten free because of the unavoidable cross-contamination with wheat that occurs during harvesting and processing. Gluten causes an autoimmune reaction, which means the body mistakenly attacks itself. The resultant damage can be physical or it can be neurological. Neurological damage includes depression, chronic fatigue, anxiety, attention deficit disorder (ADD), learning disabilities, irritability, and the inability to concentrate. What's fascinating is that these symptoms resemble emotional or behavioral dysfunction and are usually treated as such, or eliminated with medication. Yet how much is actually due to diet? There is a definite link between food, mood, and behavior that is not, as of yet, commonly understood or even explored in Western medicine. Depression is the most common symptom of gluten intolerance, yet physicians readily prescribe antidepressants and psychologists rarely suggest their patients get tested for food intolerance. The use of antidepressants may be completely unnecessary for many people, who instead need only to change their diet.

▪ Symptoms and Consequences ▪

An incredibly broad range of symptoms can indicate an intolerance to gluten. Although gastrointestinal distress has traditionally been thought to be the primary indicator, many who are gluten intolerant do not experience any digestive discomfort at all. Some may only have neurological symptoms such as depression, anxiety, and fatigue. Others may have no outward symptoms at all, while years of silent damage occur within their bodies. Many people discover their gluten intolerance only after experiencing chronic anemia, vitamin deficiencies, or osteoporosis, or by getting tested after a family member was diagnosed.

SYMPTOMS OF GLUTEN INTOLERANCE

Abdominal pain	Loss of concentration or "brain fog"
Bloating	Change in mood and disposition
Distended abdomen	Irritability
Diarrhea	Dermatitis herpetiformis
Constipation	Irregular heartbeat
Gas	Migraines
Chronic fatigue	Muscle cramps
Depression	Anemia
Anxiety	Stunted growth

Physical and mental distresses are not the only motivators to identify potential gluten intolerance. If left untreated, the consequences are serious. Continued exposure to gluten can lead to the following:

Higher risk for cancer
Increased risk for developing other autoimmune diseases,
    such as multiple sclerosis, rheumatoid arthritis,
    Hashimoto's thyroiditis, Graves' disease, Crohn's disease,
    Ulcerative colitis, and lupus
Neurological damage
Osteoporosis or bone weakness
Vitamin deficiencies because of malabsorption
Arthritis
Fibromyalgia
Miscarriage or birth defects

There is no medication for gluten intolerance. The only cure is to change your diet. By eliminating gluten completely, your physical and mental health is no longer at risk. However, this is more complicated than avoiding pizza at 2 AM or forgoing that croissant with coffee. Gluten is found in most processed and prepared foods. It is present in everything from soy sauce to canned soup. Following a gluten-free diet is far more complicated than just "not eating bread," and the strict diet must be maintained for the rest of your life in order to stay well. The demands involved in a lifestyle shift of this kind are enormous, and they can be frightening and overwhelming. When you're first diagnosed, it's hard to fully grasp all that is involved in maintaining a gluten-free diet, and it can be even more difficult to get others to comprehend the details and the severity of your condition. The following chapters explore these issues in greater depth.

▪ What Is Celiac Disease? ▪

Celiac disease is an incurable autoimmune condition; it is one specific branch of gluten intolerance. Any of the wide range of symptoms listed previously may be present in those with celiac disease, but the one consistency is that damage shows up in the small intestine. When even the smallest quantity of gluten is ingested, it triggers the body to attack itself, a process that inflames the lining of the small intestine. The small intestine is lined with villi, tiny featherlike strands that absorb the nutrients from food to fuel the body and the brain. When the intestinal lining is damaged, the villi are destroyed and unable to regenerate. Without the villi, it becomes impossible to absorb nutrients, and the individual becomes malnourished regardless of the quality or quantity of food he or she eats. It is only once gluten is eliminated from the diet and the autoimmune reaction subsides that the villi are able to regenerate.

Celiac disease is one of the most underdiagnosed conditions in the United States today. People can suffer for years before they learn the true cause. Patients are often improperly diagnosed and told their problems stem from irritable bowel syndrome, stress, or depression, or they are considered hypochondriacs. Most doctors don't test for celiac disease because, if they've heard of it at all, they've been taught that it's a rare disease. Therefore, it is rarely considered when a patient comes to them in distress.

▪ Related Conditions ▪

Along with celiac disease, there are other specific diseases that stem from gluten intolerance and can be cured or avoided by maintaining a gluten-free diet.

Dermatitis herpetiformis: Like celiac disease, dermatitis herpetiformis is a permanent autoimmune disease caused by gluten intolerance. In this case, the skin is affected as opposed to the intestine. The body reacts to gluten by causing a chronic blistering reaction on the skin. These lesions disappear when gluten is eliminated from the person's diet.

Refractory sprue: If celiac disease goes untreated for long enough, either by misdiagnosis or by not following a gluten-free diet, you can develop refractory sprue. This means your immune system no longer responds to the gluten-free diet and continual damage occurs to your intestinal lining. The villi do not have the opportunity to heal, resulting in extremely severe malabsorption. Treatment is equally severe, requiring steroids, harsh pharmaceutical therapies, and being fed through tubes.

▪ How Is Celiac Disease Diagnosed? ▪

An astounding number of general practitioners and gastroenterologists do not understand gluten intolerance or celiac disease, the seriousness of it, and its prevalence. Some don't even know the condition exists at all. Because of this, many people suffer for years before being properly diagnosed. If you have reason to believe that you may be gluten intolerant, or if a relative has learned that he or she is gluten intolerant, go to your doctor and request the proper testing. Some people have an absolutely excruciating time getting their doctors to run the simple blood tests. If your doctor refuses to run the tests, ask that he or she put it in writing and sign two copies, one for the doctor's records and one for you to keep. This tactic is more a demonstration of your rights as a patient than a solution to the issue, but it may help alter whatever the doctor's preconceptions may be. If you encounter such unfortunate behavior, or your doctor shows reluctance in running tests or discussing the possibility of gluten intolerance, do not hesitate to find a new doctor. Recommendations of knowledgeable physicians and gastroenterologists can be found through local support groups or online forums. See the Resources (page 183) for details.

Blood Tests

Blood antibody tests are the first screening tool. When your doctor tests you for gluten intolerance, these are the tests that should be performed:

Tissue Transglutaminase IgA and IgG (TTg-IgA and IgG)
Anti-Endomysial Antibodies IgA (EMA IgA)
Anti-Gliadin Antibodies IgA and IgG (AGA IgA and IgG)
Total Serum IgA (IgA Deficiency)

Blood tests are a good indicator of gluten intolerance, but they do not offer a conclusive diagnosis. In order for the antibodies to show up, you must be eating gluten regularly. However, even when there is adequate gluten in your system, tests can show a false negative or can come back with inconsistent results. Further testing via biopsy or elimination diet is quite often necessary for a conclusive answer.

Biopsy

The most respected test to determine celiac disease is a biopsy of the small intestine. This is performed by endoscopy, which is a tube that goes down your throat and takes several samples from the intestine. It's not as horrible as it sounds. You must eat gluten regularly for at least one month prior to your biopsy. The test takes samples of the small intestine and evaluates them for villi damage, so if you are not regularly ingesting gluten, the villi may heal and your intestines will look normal, resulting in a false-negative result.

It is important to choose both a gastroenterologist and a pathologist who are experienced in celiac disease. Lack of proper knowledge or experience in both the gastroenterologist who administers the biopsy and the lab that reads it can result in a false negative. Enough samples must be taken from the proper areas of the intestine to avoid misleading findings. An inexperienced pathologist may misinterpret the biopsy slides themselves, resulting in an inaccurate diagnosis. If you have doubts about who will conduct your biopsy, get in touch with local celiac support groups or check online forums for physician recommendations.

There is the potential for a negative biopsy if you have gluten intolerance that is not specifically celiac disease. As noted before, celiac disease is just one branch of gluten intolerance that happens to show gastrointestinal damage, and an intestinal biopsy is not a proper tool for diagnosis for other cases of gluten intolerance. Unfortunately, since gluten intolerance is just beginning to be well understood, there are not many specific or conclusive tests available. Blood tests and allergy tests are good indicators, but they are not by any means definitive. The elimination diet, administered by you or monitored by a nutritionist, is the best measure of diagnosis for these other cases of gluten intolerance. Those with dermatitis herpetiformis may have a biopsy performed on the affected skin.

Capsule Endoscopy

Capsule endoscopy is a new technology that offers more reliable and conclusive results than the standard biopsy. It's literally a video pill that you swallow. It transmits images during its route through your intestinal tract, taking two pictures per second for the eight hours that it's in your body. It's not yet widely available, but you should discuss this option with your gastroenterologist.

The Elimination Diet

For people with noticeable physical or neurological symptoms, the elimination diet can be an immediate and obvious test. This is how I determined my own gluten intolerance. The elimination diet entails simply removing all sources of gluten from your diet and noticing what changes take place in your body and mind. If after several days your mood, energy levels, and physical symptoms improve, there is an undeniable transformation at work that warrants your acknowledgment and consideration. If you feel significantly better without gluten, why eat it? However, many people need the authority of a medical professional to diagnose their condition in order to take it seriously. If you notice beneficial results from the elimination diet, you may choose to go off the diet, continue to eat gluten, and have the appropriate medical testing done (you *must* be consuming gluten for the tests to be accurate). I believe our bodies can provide us with every answer we need, if we choose to pay attention. This method of self-diagnosis takes diligence, awareness, and trust in yourself, and, for an accurate determination, one must be methodical and systematic. There are variables to be aware of: an additional food allergy or intolerance could mask the improvements of the gluten-free diet, you could be unknowingly consuming gluten from a hidden source, or your body could require an extended period of time to display any benefits. While most people who suffer from gluten intolerance will notice an immediate improvement in their health and well-being simply by following a gluten-free diet, specific elimination diets have been created to test for food allergies and intolerances and take these variables into account in order to ensure accurate results. Elimination diets, also called rotation diets, are simple but have very strict guidelines. If you are interested in trying an elimination diet, check out a book from the library specifically about food allergies and intolerances. Most of these books have an elimination diet outlined for you to follow. The Internet is another gold mine for this information.

▪ Dairy Intolerance ▪

It's quite common to develop an intolerance to dairy around the same time as the gluten intolerance. The dairy intolerance is often temporary, lasting about six months, until there is significant healing within your body. Your weakened digestive system is unable to properly digest the milk sugar (lactose) or the milk protein (casein). If you continue to feel physical discomfort while keeping a strict gluten-free diet, you are likely experiencing a dairy intolerance. It can be dreadfully hard to give up both wheat and dairy. In fact, losing dairy was more devastating to me than losing gluten at the time. I tried everything—Lactaid, yogurt, goat's milk—all products that contain less lactose, but to no avail. As a last desperate attempt, I bought some raw milk, and by what seemed a miracle, drank it with no problems at all. Raw milk has all of the natural enzymes intact, which help your body to digest the milk and prevent the typical reactions from occurring. Raw milk is unpasteurized and can be hard to find, as it is not legal in every state. Some states allow raw milk products to be sold in stores (check your health food stores), and some only allow it to be sold directly from the farmer, at the farm. There is absolutely nothing unsafe about raw dairy products that are produced and shipped according to the required standards. Raw milk is often organic, and because it is raw, the nutrients in the milk are intact and the protein is more easily assimilated by the body. Many varieties of divine raw cheeses are out there to explore as well.

▪ The Healing Process ▪

When foods that contain gluten are removed from your diet, healing begins immediately. The healing process varies by individual, but most people can feel a shift in their physical and mental well-being within days. It may take months, even years, to feel consistently strong and healthy and have sustained energy. Be gentle with yourself and understand that your body has been through months or years of being sick and repairing the damage doesn't happen overnight. Those with celiac disease may also be dealing with the effects of malabsorption: because of damaged villi, it's likely that you will have vitamin deficiencies as well. Making a conscious effort to eat a broad range of fresh, raw fruits and vegetables, drinking fresh, raw fruit and vegetable juices (which are easier on the digestive system), along with taking appropriate supplements, will help replenish your mineral stores.

A universal concern during the healing process is the extent of damage that is done if you accidentally consume gluten. Any time gluten is ingested, accidentally or otherwise, damage will occur. Some people have violent physical reactions to even the slightest bit of gluten, some feel "off" emotionally or have a horrible mood swing, and others have no symptoms or reactions at all. The mild nature or absence of a reaction does not mean internal damage is not occurring. An accident can be scary and miserable, but it does not set you back to the beginning. It is no fun, but not ruinous, because the impact is cumulative. Internal damage, if it is an isolated incident, is repaired quickly. Take the day off and heal. But the bottom line remains: Once you know you are gluten intolerant, you must do everything you can to avoid gluten forever.

The beauty of this condition is that it requires no drugs, no medical treatments. As soon as you stop eating gluten, you begin to heal. Your energy returns, along with clarity and joy, as you cross the threshold into radiant health.

3

A HEALTHY CHOICE
FOR EVERY BODY

Though nearly one-third of Americans are sensitive to gluten, an intolerance is not the only reason to avoid gluten. It's becoming evident that everyone may benefit from limiting their consumption of gluten-based products. Gluten cereal grains are difficult to digest, they compromise the body's ability to maintain maximum health, and they can have an adverse effect upon brain chemistry. These reactions are not limited to those with gluten intolerance; they are biological facts that affect everybody. Regardless of whether one has an intolerance, significantly decreasing the amount of gluten in the diet may likely bring enormous improvements in both health and vitality. It may be a radical suggestion, but a gluten-free lifestyle is something for everyone to explore.

Digestion requires more of our energy than any other function of the body. Wheat and dairy are two of the most difficult substances for humans to metabolize because of the nature of the proteins they contain. Protein is made up of peptide chains that are strings of amino acid; different proteins have different combinations and configurations. Gluten, the protein in wheat, and casein, the protein in milk, have certain peptides that, because of their configuration, cannot be digested by humans at all. Therefore, the amount of energy the body devotes to processing foods that contain gluten or casein is increased even further beyond the normal scope. In simplistic terms, trying to digest gluten and casein takes energy away from all the other tasks your body has: fighting disease, repairing tissue, everything down to keeping your skin soft and youthful. These peptides can also block endorphin production, the chemical the body produces to make you feel happy and good, and can interfere with proper functioning of the immune system.

Eating raw food with every meal and eliminating substances that tax the body, such as gluten (wheat products), casein (dairy products), sugar and calorie-free sugar substitutes, trans fats and hydrogenated oils, and chemicals from heavily processed foods, can actually reverse the aging process and help you overcome physical and neurological ailments. Enzymes present in raw foods aid the digestive process, so the body does not have to expend as much of its own energy on digestion. Avoiding substances that the body has difficulty processing allows energy to be directed, instead, toward general health, brain functions, and physical appearance. There is a significant indirect benefit to limiting processed foods made from refined or toxic ingredients, to choosing an apple over a croissant. The food you fill up on will likely have a higher nutrient value than processed or refined foods do, containing far more of the vitamins and minerals your body thrives on. Your energy will skyrocket, your immune system will strengthen and keep you well, and you will glow.

CNN published a report in June of 2004 stating that junk food makes up one-third of the average American's diet. Over 60 percent of Americans are overweight. The number of people with type 2 diabetes is rapidly increasing. Depression and fatigue are overwhelmingly common. Poor health is epidemic. Being forced to make drastic changes in diet and lifestyle because of a severe food intolerance can be an enormous blessing in disguise because it's so hard to choose to change your habits and dependencies when you don't feel required to do so. However, it is worth the effort. Many cultures understand that illness and disease often stem from the diet. If you feel unwell, consider the food that you eat. Drugs are available to alleviate nearly any symptom, but they don't address the damage that is being done. Many autoimmune diseases that have no cure can be improved or put into complete remission by eliminating gluten from the diet. A host of other conditions, mental and physical, can reap massive benefits by cutting out gluten, just through the pure science of energy management within the body. If your system doesn't need to constantly deal with indigestible, toxic foods, it can spend time on you. There is potential for powerful healing. So much suffering could be avoided by millions of people, without drugs and without financial strain.

Most Americans have a very difficult time imagining life without wheat, yet the majority of people in the world thrive on non-gluten grains as the staples of their diet. Millet, teff, rice, sorghum, quinoa, and corn play the leading role in cultures around the world. These foods are nutritious, inexpensive, and extremely gentle on the digestive system. Our societal addiction to gluten grains has been somewhat curbed by the current low-carb mania, but so many of our traditions and our comforts revolve around wheat-based products. Cutting out gluten does not mean you have to give up bread. It does not mean you have to live without ever having another birthday cake. It simply means replacing the flours we currently use with flours made from plants other than wheat, rye, barley, and oats. You can have your gluten-free cake and eat it too.

Wheat and gluten grains, dairy products, and sugar may be staples in the American diet and difficult to avoid, but making the choice to avoid them will bring about lasting, healthful effects that will amaze you. You'll soon find how simple it is to enjoy foods that are rich and satisfying, foods that provide you with pleasure and nutrition, foods that work with your body rather than against it. This book was designed to guide everyone toward a more healthful lifestyle, with recipes to be enjoyed by all; gluten intolerance is not a prerequisite.

4

DON'T MOVE!
YOU MIGHT BE
NEAR GLUTEN

Gluten is the second most prevalent food substance in our society, after sugar. Dangers lurk in many common diet staples, and while learning to identify hidden gluten is a skill that may seem difficult and complicated, it will soon become second nature. In addition to the obvious, gluten is found in countless products ranging from soy milk to enchilada sauce. The following pages offer lists of foods that are safe, foods that contain gluten, and the numerous foods and ingredients that are questionable. These lists are helpful, but avoiding gluten is not quite that simple. There are other issues to understand in order to stay safe and healthy.

▪ Reading Labels ▪

If you want anything that comes from a package, from raw meat to salad dressing to chocolate chips, you must read the entire list of ingredients before you eat it. It becomes a habit quite quickly, though initially it makes sense to carry a list of the ingredients to beware of. Many common additives are derived from gluten, and gluten-based ingredients are often used as fillers. Some ingredients can be made from gluten sources *or* gluten-free sources. If the product in question contains any of these ingredients, you must call the manufacturer to determine if the product is truly gluten free.

▪ Calling Food and Drug Companies ▪

To determine the source of ambiguous ingredients, or to understand the production environment (see "Cross-Contamination," below), you must call the manufacturer directly. The appropriate phone number can be found on the packaging material of the product. It makes sense to make a list of the products you use regularly and set aside an afternoon to make all the necessary phone calls in one fell swoop.

Key Questions to Ask Manufacturers

➤ Do any of the ingredients used in this product contain gluten?
➤ Are any third-party ingredients used that the manufacturer of the product cannot vouch for?
➤ Does the production facility pose a threat for cross-contamination?
➤ Are gluten-containing items produced in the same facility? On the same lines?
➤ What precautions against cross-contamination does the manufacturer take?
➤ What are their testing procedures?

You can also reference the manufacturer's Web site to check the gluten-free status of many products, since companies often list nutritional data and allergen information online. This may not, however, clear up the question of cross-contamination during production. Another option, in a pinch, is to search the archives of online forums for information on a particular product. Be aware, though, that this can be risky. The information may not be accurate or it may not be current—companies change their recipes, even in the most enduring products; some products even have different ingredients depending on where they are produced and sold.

▪ Cross-Contamination ▪

The dangers of cross-contamination are serious and widespread, and represent one of the most difficult and irritating aspects of maintaining a gluten-free diet. The fact that a product has gluten-free ingredients does not necessarily mean that it is safe. Cross-contamination turns food that should be safe into toxic accidents waiting to happen. The following are important things to know about the cross-contamination that can occur during food production, preparation, and cooking.

Cross-Contamination during Production:
➤ Puffed cereals and chips have a high risk for cross-contamination if the manufacturer does not take precautions. Puffing creates large quantities of

dust, and if wheat is being puffed near gluten-free products, the gluten-free items can get covered in wheat dust.

➤ If gluten and gluten-free products are produced on the same lines using the same machinery, cross-contamination can occur via leftover residue.

➤ Another indicator of cross-contamination is if a large number of other gluten-intolerant people have had reactions to particular "gluten-free" products. The final decision is always yours to make, but it can be helpful to learn what the experiences of others have been. See the Resources chapter for support groups and online forums.

➤ Some companies have designated gluten-free facilities. This is ideal.

Cross-Contamination during Preparation and Cooking:

➤ *Frying Oils:* When breaded products are fried, bits of the bread batter remain in the oil, like crumbs. These bits can then stick to other foods that are cooked in the same oil. For example, if french fries are fried in oil that is also used for frying breaded items, it is more than likely the fries will be contaminated with bits of residual flour batter.

➤ *Fillers:* Gluten is often used as a filler in what would seem to be gluten-free food. For example, flour is often used as a binder in hamburger patties.

➤ *Contaminated Grill or Griddle:* If your meal is cooked on a grill or griddle that has not been well cleaned after gluten food was cooked there, you are in danger of cross-contamination. This can be in the form of crumbs from bread products or residue from marinades that contain soy sauce.

➤ *Other:* Ice-cream shops are yet another example of potential cross-contamination, in this instance from broken cone shards in the ice cream.

This all sounds a bit crazy, but it's important to know. It's also important not to go off the deep end of paranoia and refuse to eat anything for fear of contamination. You'll soon be an expert at choosing the right foods to maintain your health.

■ ■ ■

FOODS THAT CONTAIN GLUTEN

Barley	Licorice	Rye
Barley malt	Malt	Seitan
Beer	Malt flavoring	Semolina
Bulgur	Malt syrup	Shoyu
Couscous	Malt vinegar	Soy sauce
Durum	Maltose	Spelt
Einkorn	Nama shoyu	Triticale
Farina	Oats	Wheat
Graham	Oat flour	Wheat germ
Kamut	Pearl barley	Wheat starch

GLUTEN-FREE FOODS

Agar-agar	Dextrose	Quinoa flour
Alcohol and spirits	Glutamine	Rice
Amaranth	Glutinous rice	Rice flour
Amaranth flour	Kasha	Sorghum
Arabic gum	Maltodextrin	Sorghum flour
Arrowroot	Maltitol	Soy
Bean flours	Masa harina	Soy flour
Buckwheat	Millet	Succotash
Buckwheat flour	Millet flour	Tapioca
Cassava	Milo	Tapioca flour
Cellulose	Milo flour	Teff
Champagne	Nut flours	Teff flour
Corn	Polenta	Vinegar: rice, white, cider,
Cornmeal	Potato	distilled, balsamic, wine
Cornstarch	Potato flour	Wild rice
Corn flour	Potato starch flour	Wine
Corn syrup	Quinoa	Xanthan gum

POTENTIAL FOOD HAZARDS

You should be especially wary of the foods listed below. Many people assume these are gluten-free foods and often that is wrong. Read labels carefully to determine if the product is safe, and call the company directly if you have any doubts.

Alcohol and spirits	Marinades	Soba noodles
Birth control pills	Miso	Soups
Corn and rice cereals	Over-the-counter drugs	Soy milk
Communion wafers	Potato chips	Spices
Enriched or fortified rice	Prescription medicines	Tamari sauce
Flavored coffee	Processed meat products	Teas
Gravies and sauces	Processed tofu products	Vegetable cooking spray
Imitation seafood	Seasoned raw meats	Vitamins

The following ingredients are commonly found in processed foods and can either be made from wheat or barley, and therefore contain gluten, or they can be made from rice, potatoes, corn, or tapioca, all of which are safe. When you see any of the ingredients listed, call the manufacturer to determine if that ingredient was derived from a gluten-free source.

Artificial color	Modified food starch
Artificial flavors	Modified starch
Brown rice syrup	Mono- and diglycerides
Caramel color	Natural flavors
Dextrin	Rice malt
Food starch	Rice syrup
Hydrolyzed vegetable protein (HVP)	Textured vegetable protein (TVP)
Hydrolyzed plant protein (HPP)	Vegetable starch

FOOD GLOSSARY

Reading food labels can seem like learning a new language. Here is a further explanation of some of the more confusing terms.

Alcohol and vinegar: The distillation process removes gluten; however, flavoring added after distillation may contain gluten. Though there has been much debate over this topic, vinegar is gluten free with the exception of malt vinegar. Apple cider, balsamic, distilled, white, and wine vinegar are all safe, unless, of course, they have added flavorings that contain gluten.

Dextrin: Usually made from corn but may be made from wheat and therefore may contain gluten.

Dextrose: Dextrose is always made from corn and is gluten free.

Glutinous rice: Another name for sticky rice, glutinous rice does not contain gluten.

Imitation seafood: Wheat flour is often used as a binder in imitation seafood and therefore could contain gluten. Also, be aware that restaurants may mix fresh seafood with imitation seafood, thereby causing contamination. Always ask the server if this is practiced.

Kasha: Kasha is roasted buckwheat kernels and is gluten free.

Maltitol: This is a sugar alcohol that does not contain malt or gluten, despite its name.

Maltodextrin: Made from corn or potato, maltodextrin is gluten free.

Milo: Another name for sorghum, milo is gluten free.

Oats and oat flour: Oats do not inherently contain gluten; however, they are not safe because of unavoidable cross-contamination with wheat during harvesting and processing.

Polenta: A traditional, slow-cooked gluten-free cornmeal dish, polenta can be baked, fried, grilled, or cooked as a pudding.

Raw meat: I got very sick after buying ground turkey, thinking it was undoubtedly gluten free, when in fact it had been seasoned with a product containing gluten. Be aware of added seasonings and spices.

Rice syrup and brown rice syrup: Frequently made with added barley, these syrups may therefore contain gluten.

Spices: Wheat flour may be used to prevent spices from clumping, and may not be listed on the ingredient list.

Teas: Some teas, primarily the "mock coffee" teas, contain barley or flavorings that contain gluten.

Gluten-free Flours

Arrowroot: A very fine flour that is a good thickening agent, arrowroot is similar to cornstarch but reacts differently to heat and certain ingredients.

Bean flours: Open for you to experiment with; I've never used them. They impart a strong bean flavor to the finished product. Bean flour also has the same effect on your body as beans do.

Buckwheat: Buckwheat has nothing to do with wheat. It is not a grain but rather a plant related to rhubarb. This nutritious food contains all eight essential amino acids, delivering high-quality protein along with good amounts of minerals and dietary fiber.

Corn flour: Finely ground corn, corn flour has a true flour texture with the taste of corn.

Cornmeal: Coarsely ground corn, this is available in yellow and blue varieties. The blue turns food purple, which is fun.

Cornstarch: This is a very fine flour that is used primarily as a thickener.

Masa harina: Another corn flour, masa harina is used in authentic Mexican dishes.

Millet flour: This whole-grain flour is quite nutritious and considered the most easily digestible.

Nut flours: These are really expensive! Make your own for almost half the price by grinding nuts in the blender or coffee grinder.

Rice flour: I don't use rice flour in this book, though it is a conventional staple of gluten-free cooking. I stopped using rice flour for several reasons: Rice flour is grainy, which imparts an odd texture to the finished product; white rice flour has very little nutritional value; sweet rice flour has a smooth texture, but anecdotal data shows that this product is commonly cross-contaminated.

■ ■ ■

Sorghum: Also known as milo flour or jowar, this flour has been used as a staple in Africa and India for thousands of years. High in antioxidants and very nutritious, sorghum is a member of the grass family.

Soy flour: Soy flour is high in protein and also high in fat, for a flour. It also has great flavor. Soy flour gives off an odd smell when you are mixing it in batter, but this vanishes when it is cooked.

Tapioca flour: This is another very fine flour without much nutrition. It does add chewiness to recipes.

Teff flour: Because this flour is whole grain, it is dense in nutrients and high in protein and fiber. Teff has a rich savory flavor and is a staple of Ethiopian cuisine.

Xanthan gum: An essential ingredient in gluten-free baking, xanthan gum mimics the puff and fluff of gluten.

5

MAKING THE
TRANSITION

The transition into a gluten-free lifestyle can be overwhelming on many levels. In addition to learning completely new dietary guidelines, you must deal with various difficulties that are much more subtle and complex. The level of responsibility that is required to stay healthy is daunting. A complete restructuring your life, your time, your priorities, even your interactions with others becomes necessary.

Food is more than just fuel; it has tremendous emotional significance. It is a way in which we connect with our past and with the people in our lives. Many memories and emotions are attached to certain foods; they represent traditions, special occasions, nostalgic moments. It is hard to sever those ties. What makes it easier is to begin to create new moments, new memories, and new traditions to imbue your gluten-free life.

Meanwhile, prepare for emotions that may surface during this transition—anger, hurt, and confusion. You have every right to mourn what you've lost. Just don't get bitter. You can choose to feel like this has happened *to* you, or that it has happened *for* you. The most potent tool you have to affect your healing is the way in which you think about your situation.

This transition is just that: a transition. Think of it this way: New habits form after 21 steady days of practice. What seems overwhelming will soon become second nature, and the difficulties that affect you now may disappear sooner than you think.

■ ■ ■

■ Social Issues ■

For many, the most difficult aspect of dealing with gluten intolerance is not the restricted diet, but rather the social awkwardness that can result. Most of our social gatherings revolve around food: family and business, traditions and celebrations, relationships and romance. Sharing meals with others is one of the few ways we connect in our hectic society, and that ritual is now disrupted by worry, inconvenience, or embarrassment. Since gluten is so pervasive, participating in these occasions while avoiding potentially dangerous food becomes a complicated task. It can create a feeling of isolation, especially if others assume by your behavior that you are an outlandishly picky eater, that you have an eating disorder, or that you are crazy.

Dining at restaurants, at friend's homes, or with relatives all present their own challenges. There are a million things to be aware of, from both a technical standpoint and an emotional one. It can be stressful, irritating, even devastating. However, these situations present you with opportunities to be creative, to instigate healing, to invent fun and wonderful ways to connect with the people you care about that don't necessarily involve food. Through it all, it is important to remember that your peace, your health, and your happiness are your responsibility.

■ Restaurants ■

Eating out is always risky. There are so many possible dangers and potential problems. Restaurant kitchens are extremely busy, and many people are involved in the creation of your meal. Most people are unaware of the requirements of the gluten-free diet—the minutiae that must be considered—and it is ridiculous to expect the people preparing your food to grasp all the details. Even after you clearly explain how important it is that there be no wheat, flour, or ingredients that contain gluten, such as soy sauce, used in the preparation of your food, you never truly know if your meal is safe to eat. Servers or cooks may not fully understand what your requirements are, or they may not take it seriously, equating it with a trendy weight-loss diet. There is always the potential for cross-contamination via grills, pans, and utensils. There is also the potential for naive mistakes to occur, such as simmering pasta water being used to heat your "plain" vegetables. A further consideration is determining whether gluten is contained in any of the products that are used as ingredients in what is being made. This is an issue down to your morning coffee—any soy latte drinkers should be aware that certain brands of soy milk are not gluten free.

Slowly, the number of restaurants that understand gluten intolerance and promote gluten-free dining is growing. Some are independents; some are chains. Search online discussion groups or contact local support groups for recommendations for gluten-free-friendly restaurants in your area. If you have a relationship with a chef, server, or owner of a restaurant, you can introduce the topic. If you have a favorite restaurant that you don't want to "lose," suggest that gluten-free-friendly dining is a niche waiting to be filled. By establishing relationships within a restaurant, you can feel safe because they know you, understand your needs, and will accommodate you.

TIPS FOR DINING OUT SAFELY

■ Describe the situation as a medical condition or a severe food allergy so it is more likely to be taken seriously.

■ Explain your situation directly to the manager as well as the server.

■ If you consistently have problems in restaurants, have a man do the talking. It is unfortunate that, generally speaking, men are still taken more seriously than women, considered more authoritative, and are more intimidating if a mistake is made.

■ Print out a restaurant card to give to your server.*

■ Tell the server that all bread products must be kept away from your food.

■ Order plain food (i.e., vegetables, chicken breast, baked potato), and ask that no seasonings or sauces be used.

■ Peruse the menu for "safe" items within each meal and put together your own special à la carte mishmash.

■ Order a lovely, entree-sized salad. Ask for a special salad to be put together if what you have in mind is not on the menu. Specify raw ingredients, no croutons, and a simple oil and vinegar dressing, though if you request avocado, you won't even need dressing.

■ Eat beforehand, and just order a drink or a small salad at the restaurant.

■ Do not hesitate to send food back if it is wrong, and explain that it must be redone from scratch to prevent contamination.

■ Call the restaurant ahead of time to alert them of your reservation, explain your condition, and make arrangements for menu substitutions or gluten-free alterations.

■ Trust. A meal where you are worried the whole time is not enjoyable.

* Restaurant dining cards can be downloaded from www.glutenfreerestaurants.org. These can be given to your server to give to the chef. They look "official," and demand an extra step in acknowledging the issue, but they still in no way ensure that your food will be safe.

Because of the range of concerns, most people cut back on the frequency with which they dine out after learning of their gluten intolerance. So much of our time with others, however, happens in restaurants, and there is really no reason to vanish from your social scene. You can do it without compromising your health, with a little flexibility and honesty. The emphasis when going out with others is on enjoying one another. Allowing your gluten intolerance to keep you from your life will only make your transition longer and more difficult.

■ Dining with Relatives and Friends ■

Sharing a meal at the home of a friend or relative brings up its own set of issues to contend with. You cannot expect the average person to comprehend the nuances of what gluten free means. There is so much to grasp, so many "normal" ingredients where gluten can hide, and so many ways to inadvertently make a mistake that it can be unrealistic to trust any meal that you don't prepare yourself. This does not mean you need to stay at home.

Here are some ways to stay in the fun and also stay safe:

➤ Bring a dish to share.
➤ Offer to help out in the kitchen during preparation, so in fact you can oversee what goes on.
➤ Eat beforehand, nibble on veggies, and drink those eight glasses of water you're supposed to get each day while everyone else eats.
➤ Remember that everyone is there for the camaraderie, not the food. Enjoy your time.

In addition to navigating the technicalities of the meal, dining with friends, and, in particular, family, can often bring intense feelings into play. Hopefully, most of the people in your life will be understanding and supportive, and do what they can to make you feel comfortable, safe, and loved. However, it can seem like other people in your life are trying to kill you. Such individuals can add a very taxing dimension to everything that you are already dealing with. There is a fine line between ignorance and insensitivity. Just keep reminding yourself that it's hard, if not impossible, for someone who is not gluten intolerant to comprehend the intricacies: the innumerable hiding places of gluten, what it is like to live with restrictions, the way an accidental mishap that can wipe you out, and the enormous stress you are under at the beginning.

An astounding number of conflicts occur between family members, usually at holidays, over food, over gluten intolerance, over gluten-free food, or any variation on the theme. Holidays and celebrations can seem more centered on food and food traditions than being with loved ones and doing things together. If people want you to be involved in an occasion, then some concessions have to be made to ensure your safety and your health. By the same token, your expectations of others cannot be so high that they are unattainable.

Here are some points to remember:

➤ Food doesn't define the spirit of holiday, or any other day.
➤ Maintaining a gluten-free diet is a medical necessity. There is no reason to go off the gluten-free diet to appease anyone.
➤ Your life and your health are your priority, and you can be faithful to this and polite to others at the same time.
➤ Traditions evolve and change. Initiate something new, special, and meaningful.

Some ways to address animosity you may be confronted with include:

➤ Arrive as the meal is ending.
➤ Bring your own gorgeous gluten-free meal. This can make your separateness obvious and instigate an open discussion if one needs to happen.
➤ Bring enough to share, so others see that gluten-free food tastes as good, if not better, than their food.
➤ Only take part in events that don't revolve around food.
➤ Change your expectations of people.

You must decide what is right for you, and this may change as time goes by. Maintaining an awareness of your body and self is empowering and will help you make educated choices. In the end, it's up to you to determine what is harmful, both physically and emotionally, and to keep yourself away from those environments.

▪ Eating at Formal Engagements ▪

Everyone will have their own opinion about how to deal with attending weddings and other formal parties. If the occasion is to celebrate an important step in someone else's life, I think it is out of place to bring up your dietary needs to the host or hostess, unless asked. It is very easy to discreetly bring a simple meal for yourself to eat in lieu of what is being catered. If people around you wonder what you are doing, use the opportunity to explain your condition. There are so many people who are dealing with the consequences of gluten intolerance and are not diagnosed, you just may shed light on another's suffering.

Dates have the potential to be very awkward—I would never want to delve into this topic with some cutie I barely knew. Here's another opportunity for you to be creative about the situation and make life a thrill. Consider how much time and money is spent on the standard dinner and a movie. Think of all the thousands of things you can do in that amount of time with that amount of money. The possibilities are endless. These dates will be memorable even if your date is not.

▨ The Big Picture ▨

Often, an illness will present itself in tandem with another, nonphysical issue, one that may be spiritual or emotional. Through dealing with the physical ailment, you are given the opportunity to address and overcome an issue in your internal life. I mention this because living with gluten intolerance is an enormous challenge. It can be easier and more rewarding if you see what is going on in the larger picture and view the uncomfortable situations, the painful situations, the embarrassing situations, and the angering situations as a hologram, in a way. They exist to present you with opportunities for you to make a choice about how you will deal with them and how you will be affected by them. Inevitably, your psyche will incorporate these choices into the person you are becoming.

Issues you may be dealing with include the following:

> *Willpower:* How to relinquish foods that are steeped in tradition and nostalgia and ceremony.
> *Patience:* How to deal gently yet firmly with people who simply don't understand your condition, who are not malicious, merely ignorant.
> *Composure:* Not be bothered by scorn or sarcasm from people who don't take you seriously—in other words, if it's not being cured by a pill, it's not a real illness.
> *Creativity:* How to use your imagination to initiate new traditions. How to create new ways to share life with the people you care about that don't necessarily revolve around food.
> *Speaking up:* How to be authoritative about to your needs. How to stand up for yourself with family, friends, or business associates.
> *Slowing down:* How to dedicate time to prepare your meals and allow yourself to use that time to separate from the rest of your day.

➤ *Speaking out:* How to share your experience in a way that is constructive and helpful to others.

➤ *Initiating a rapport with your own body:* How to appreciate what your body is capable of, pay attention to what it tells you, and not to ignore its needs.

➤ *Taking charge:* Coming to terms with the fact that you're the only one who can rescue yourself from this illness.

➤ *Getting over it:* How to stop considering yourself ill or disadvantaged. You'll reach this point only when you become grateful for what has happened because you know that as a result, you have gained far more than you lost.

▪ Being Healthy ▪

Health is a choice. After experiencing the awful repercussions of malabsorption, you gain an understanding of the importance of a healthy and balanced diet. Food becomes more than just "food." Nutritious food represents the fuel we need to live well and feel wonderful. We can use this awareness to our benefit and see the dimensions of everything we choose to put into our body.

When you eat prepared foods, risk is inevitable. Processed foods often contain hidden gluten, and these products are generally stripped of their nutrients and contain excessive sugar, chemicals, and trans fats. Eliminating such foods means less worry and greater health. This is an opportunity for you to raise your standards for what you choose to put into your body.

Organic produce and free-range meats are more expensive than conventional products, which can be a huge issue when shopping. However, what you put into your body is one of the most important things you can spend your money on. Pesticides, chemicals, and additives will weaken your system and destroy you from the inside out.

Fresh produce is always the most nutritious choice. Canned and frozen fruits and vegetables have undergone processing that strips them of some of their intrinsic healthful properties: enzymes, nutrients, and antioxidants. However, canned and frozen items are very convenient, and it is far better to eat frozen or canned fruits and vegetables than to not eat them at all.

Microwaving vegetables causes them to lose the majority of their antioxidants and other cancer-fighting compounds. To avoid this, steam, roast, sauté, or enjoy them raw.

▪ ▪ ▪

■ Take Care of the Earth ■
While Taking Care of Yourself

When you start cooking a lot, you start shopping a lot. With this comes a new set of responsibilities and considerations to be aware of. All are simple and easy, but have lasting effects on our Earth. Keep the following in mind:

➤ Walk to the store if or when you can.
➤ Reuse shopping bags.
➤ Recycle everything! Cardboard and paper packaging, cans, bottles, tinfoil, even plastic shopping bags. Most grocery stores have a collection area for recycling plastic grocery bags; if yours doesn't, ask them to start one.
➤ Use cloth dish towels and save paper towels for the really icky messes.
➤ Buy in bulk! Many health food stores have a bulk section, with bins of spices and rices and all sorts of goodies. This is so much cheaper and it saves so much packaging. And when you buy in bulk, you can get as much, or as little, as you like.
➤ Use biodegradable cleaning products. Chemicals are bad for you and the world.
➤ Buy organic whenever you can.
➤ Eat happy, healthy animals: free-range, organic, cage-free, and antibiotic-free meat and eggs.
➤ Support local farmers. The food is fresher and fewer resources are used in transportation.

■ Starting to Cook ■

Cooking can seem like a terrifying, time-consuming, and nerve-racking proposition to a beginner. When I first started to cook, the stress and pressure that came along with learning was very intense, and I was never sure if the time and money I put into a dish would result in anything edible by the time I was done. It can be difficult to find the proper flours, basic cooking equipment can be costly, and setting up a gluten-free environment if you live with other people can be complicated.

However, cooking is now an unavoidable part of your life. Unless you can hire a personal chef, you will have to cook. Accepting this fact can help turn the time you spend in the kitchen from a stressful irritation to something wonderful. You're stuck there, so you might as well try to enjoy it. Use it as a time to daydream, a respite from the rest of life. Chopping vegetables can become a meditation.

The fact that I have written a cookbook makes me wonder if I am living in some sort of parallel universe. Had I been told two years ago this was in my future, I would have laughed and declared it impossible. But nothing is impossible, and cooking has actually become easy and even fun (though I am still loath to admit that).

Cooking does not need to be a sentence. Celebrate the freedom you have. Make alterations. Add or substitute ingredients with what you have around or with your favorite foods. Don't be afraid to experiment. Sometimes improvisations can turn out awful, but success is much more common. Your dishes will be unique and special—your own creations.

6

KITCHEN ESSENTIALS

Until recently, I used my oven for storage and my only dishes were an old tin pie pan that I used as a plate and fairy-sized ceramic bowls made by my little sister. Much has changed. When cooking becomes part of your daily routine, life becomes easier if you swallow your pride and invest in the equipment that will help you. When you begin your foray into cooking, the following is what you will need.

Essential Equipment
    Medium saucepan with lid
    Large frying pan with lid
        Note: Chef's pans are a hybrid of a saucepan and a frying pan—they are
        large, lidded, and can be used in circumstances that call for either.
    Large stockpot with lid
    Steamer basket that fits one of the pots
    Large mixing bowl
    Measuring cups
    Measuring spoons
    Chef's knife, for chopping
    Serrated knife, for slicing
    Large wooden spoon
    Garlic press
    Can opener
    Cutting board
    Cookie sheet with raised edges
    8-x-8-inch baking dish

8½-x-4½-x-2½-inch loaf pan
Muffin pan (either one 12-muffin pan or two 6-muffin pans)
Blender

Convenient but Not Essential

Spatula
Ladle
Ramekins
Sieve
Cheese grater
Colander
Lettuce spinner
More knives
More pots, pans, and mixing bowls
Baking dishes of different sizes and shapes
Handheld mixer
Mandoline (see page 145 for more information)
Food processor

Essential Spices

Don't be daunted by the rows of spices at the store, or by their cost. You only need to start with a few to add fabulous and diverse flavor to your meals. Health food stores often sell herbs and spices in bulk, so you can just buy what you need and add to your collection bit by bit.

Sea salt	Rosemary
Black pepper	Dill
Cumin	Curry
Cayenne	Coriander
Cinnamon	Cloves
Ginger	Nutmeg

■ Measurement Conversions, ■ Substitutions, and Storage Tips

Measurement Conversions

Volume
3 teaspoons = 1 tablespoon
4 tablespoons = ¼ cup
8 tablespoons = ½ cup
1 ounce = 2 tablespoons
2 ounces = ¼ cup
4 ounces = ½ cup
5 ounces = ⅔ cup
6 ounces = ¾ cup
8 ounces = 1 cup
12 ounces = 1½ cups
16 ounces = 2 cups
2 cups = 1 pint
2 pints = 1 quart
4 quarts = 1 gallon

Weight
4 ounces = ¼ pound
5 ounces = ⅓ pound
8 ounces = ½ pound
12 ounces = ¾ pound
16 ounces = 1 pound

Substitutions

Sweeteners
Each of the following sweeteners has its own unique flavor and characteristics, but they can easily be substituted for one another. Honey and agave nectar are both sweeter than sugar. If you're substituting either one for white sugar in a baking recipe, use two-thirds of what the recipe calls for. You may need to use less liquid or more flour in the recipe to achieve the proper consistency. Sucralose, aka Splenda, is made from sugar, but it has been chemically altered and is actually a chemical substance. I do not recommend it.

Honey
Agave nectar
Maple syrup
Brown sugar
Granulated sugar (refined sugar)

Milks

You can substitute any of these milks directly, based on your preference.

Almond milk
Soy milk — ? SEE PAGE 23
Rice milk
Cow's milk

Fats

2 egg whites = 1 egg
Using egg whites maintains the protein while cutting the fat content.

3 tablespoons water + 1 tablespoon flaxseed meal = 1 egg
Flaxseed contains slightly less fat than eggs; this is more applicable to vegans.

Applesauce = butter or oil
When baking, substitute 50 to 100 percent of the butter or oil with an equal amount of applesauce to reduce the fat in a recipe.

Food Storage

Generally, leftovers can be kept in the refrigerator for three to five days. Date your containers to make life easy.

Other Storage Times to Note:

Uncooked meat: 3 to 5 days in fridge, 6 months in freezer
Uncooked poultry: 1 to 2 days in fridge, 9 months in freezer
Uncooked fish: 1 to 2 days in fridge, 5 months in freezer
Uncooked shrimp: 2 to 3 days in fridge, 4 months in freezer
Cooked meat: 3 to 4 days in fridge, 2 months in freezer
Cooked poultry: 3 to 4 days in fridge, 4 months in freezer
Cooked fish: 3 to 4 days in fridge, 3 months in freezer

Cooked shrimp: 3 to 4 days in fridge, 3 months in freezer

Soup: 4 to 5 days in fridge, 3 months in freezer

Hard-boiled eggs: 1 week in fridge

Shelled nuts: 1 month in cupboard, 9 months in freezer

Flours: 3 months in refrigerator or cool, dry cupboard

Grains: 3 to 6 months in refrigerator or cool, dry cupboard

Frozen Food

Put frozen items in the fridge to thaw. Be aware that thawing food has a tendency to drip. For a faster method, put the frozen item in a ziplock bag and submerge in cold water. If you will be cooking or eating the food immediately, it can be thawed in a microwave or on the stove.

7

EXCURSIONS
AND ADVENTURES

Cooking may be an inescapable part of your life now, but there are plenty of ways to make it more fun.

▪ The Farmers' Market ▪

I cannot sing enough praise about farmers' markets. They provide a wonderful way to shop for produce and the benefits are abundant. Farmers' markets are beautiful. Crates of gorgeous, ripe fruits and vegetables overwhelm your senses. Vendors give out samples of their produce, share their immense knowledge, and friendships are easy to form, for camaraderie at the market is as natural and pure as the produce. Along with whatever fruits and vegetables are in season, you can often find farmers selling eggs, meat, fish, nuts, mushrooms, honey, dairy products, and baked goods. Prices at farmers' markets are significantly lower than at grocery stores, and you know the produce is fresh and was farmed locally. Supporting local farmers has obvious economical benefits, but it also benefits the environment because fewer resources (energy and gasoline) are used to transport local produce than is required by produce that is shipped great distances. I urge everyone to explore their local farmers' market and turn shopping from a chore into a sense-sational outing.

Most cities host at least one farmers' market. To find the farmer's market nearest you, call your local visitor's bureau or chamber of commerce, or you can search for information online.

Online listings vary in their accuracy and scope, but some helpful sites include the following:

www.ams.usda.gov
www.localharvest.org
www.openair.org/opair/twebmar.html
www.cafarmersmarkets.com (in California)
www.cenyc.org (in New York City and boroughs)

▪ The Herb Garden ▪

Even if you have no time, no outdoor space, or no success with plants, herbs are easy to grow. Having fresh herbs to add to your cooking is such a treat, and plants make life more beautiful. Herbs have long been used for their nutritive properties, while their flavor will enhance any dish. Herb plants are inexpensive to buy, or you can start them from seeds, as they grow quickly.

If you buy small plants, transplant them to a slightly larger pot so they have room to grow. Plant seeds according to the directions on the seed packet, and use an all-purpose soil mix. You can stay low budget by cutting 2-liter bottles in half and using them as pots. Whatever you decide to use as a pot, be sure to poke holes in the bottom for water drainage. Keep the plants on a sunny windowsill or on a shelf or table that gets lots of sun, as they like as much sunlight as possible. If there is nowhere to put potted plants, you can use a hanging basket. The key to happy herbs is to never overwater them. The more you cut from your plant, the more it will grow, though harvesting more than a third of the plant at one time may cause it to die.

Fresh herbs are a wonderful addition to any dish, or they can be dried to use down the road. Dry herbs by hanging the stems upside down from string or clothespins, or lay them flat on a rack or cookie sheet to dry in the oven. Keep the oven off, but turn on the oven light for warmth. Store dried herbs in a glass jar.

EASY HERBS TO GROW

Basil	Mint
Chives	Parsley
Lemon balm	Thyme

▪ **Sprouting** ▪

Sprouting is like having a little garden in a jar. Sprouts are a wonderful addition to any diet, and it is so easy and inexpensive to grow your own sprouts. Loaded with nutrients and amino acids, they are filling and low in fat. Alfalfa sprouts and mung bean sprouts are the most common, but you can also grow pea sprouts, broccoli sprouts, or adzuki bean sprouts, all in a jar on your countertop. Sprouts are great tossed in salads, and pea sprouts are so delicious I eat them on their own with a sprinkling of sea salt and a drizzle of olive oil.

There are four basic steps to sprouting: soak the seeds in water, drain the water, rinse the seeds twice a day, and eat the sprouts.

All you need to sprout are quart-size mason jars with screw-top lids (or reusable pasta sauce jars), cheesecloth, rubber bands, and your chosen seeds, which you can find in the bulk section of most health food stores. Then just use the directions that follow.

How to Sprout

1. Put the seeds in a jar, according to the guidelines that follow.

2. Cut a square of cheesecloth, four layers thick, that is slightly larger than the opening of the jar. Secure the cheesecloth over the opening of the jar, using the metal screw-ring that came with the mason jar or a sturdy rubber band. (The cheesecloth allows you to fill and drain the jar without losing the seeds and also allows air to circulate with the seeds.)

3. Fill the jar with water and pour it out a few times to rinse the seeds, then fill with water and leave the seeds to soak for the proper length of time according to the guidelines that follow.

4. Once the seeds have soaked, pour out the water. Be sure to drain the water completely; otherwise, the seeds can rot. You can shake the jar a little to drain it or leave it sitting at an angle, cheesecloth-side down.

5. Rinse the seeds twice a day for the duration of the sprouting time by filling the jar with water and pouring it directly out. This keeps the seeds moist. Soon the seeds will begin to sprout and grow little tails! So cute.

6. Grow them for the proper length of time, according to the following guidelines. Store in an airtight container in the fridge for up to five days.

SPROUTING GUIDELINES

Adzuki bean: Soak ½ cup of adzuki beans for 12 hours; sprout for 3 to 5 days.

Alfalfa: Soak 2 tablespoons of alfalfa seeds for 5 to 8 hours; sprout for 4 to 5 days.

Broccoli seed: Soak 2 tablespoons of broccoli seeds for 8 hours; sprout for 3 to 4 days.

Mung bean: Soak 1 cup of mung beans for 8 hours; sprout for 4 to 5 days.

Peas: Soak 1 cup of dried green peas for 8 hours; sprout for 2 to 3 days.

TWO

The Recipes

BREAKFAST AND BRUNCH

||||||||||||||

Though mornings can be hectic,
breakfast shouldn't be.
The following recipes offer easy and delicious
ways to start your day off right.

Hot Cakes

When you crave something fluffy and light, whip up a batch of these fantastic pancakes.

PREP: 6 minutes

COOKING: 3 minutes per pancake

TOTAL TIME: Not very long

YIELD: 10 pancakes

¾ cup plain soy milk
4 egg whites
2 tablespoons applesauce
½ cup sorghum flour
½ cup millet flour
1 tablespoon arrowroot
1½ teaspoons sugar
1½ teaspoons baking powder
½ teaspoon xanthan gum

1. Put the soy milk, egg whites, and applesauce in a blender and blend well.
2. Add the sorghum flour, millet flour, arrowroot, sugar, baking powder, and xanthan gum to the blender and blend briefly. Scrape down the sides with a spatula and briefly blend again.
3. Pour batter into a frying pan that has been warmed over medium heat.
4. Flip to cook both sides, about 2 to 3 minutes total.
5. Drench with butter and maple syrup, spread with jam, or just eat plain.

Tasty Variations

Stir in a cup of fresh blueberries—add to the batter once it is mixed.

Spice up these pancakes with cardamom—add ¼ teaspoon with the other dry ingredients.

Try flaxseed meal for some nutty nutrition—add 2 tablespoons with the dry ingredients.

Huevos Rancheros

These are simple enough to fix on a busy morning, yet taste like you're breakfasting at a sidewalk café.

PREP: 5 minutes

COOKING: 7 minutes

TOTAL TIME: 10 minutes

YIELD: 2

2–4 eggs
1 15-ounce can black beans
1 4-ounce can mild green chilies
Dash hot sauce, if desired
¼ cup grated cheddar or Monterey Jack
    cheese
2 corn tortillas
1 tomato

1. Prepare the eggs according to the Easiest Eggs recipe (see page 53).
2. While the eggs are cooking, put the black beans in a bowl with 2 tablespoons of green chilies. Microwave on high for about 15 seconds, or until heated through, and season with hot sauce.
3. Put a layer of cheese on each corn tortilla and place them on a square of tinfoil. Heat them under the oven broiler for 1 to 2 minutes to melt the cheese and crisp the tortillas. In the meantime, chop the tomato.
4. Put a cheese tortilla on a plate and cover with the bean and chili mixture. Place an egg, once it has cooked, on the beans, and top with chopped tomato. Repeat for the second portion. *Voilà!* Or, rather, *Olé!*

Cinnamon Rolls

Gooey but not too sweet, these cinnamon rolls are a lovely treat. They are a bit of a time investment but definitely worth it. Make a double batch and freeze the extras to reheat in the oven or microwave whenever the mood hits.

PREP: 25 minutes

RISE: 1½ hours

COOKING: 15 minutes

TOTAL TIME: 2 hours, 10 minutes

YIELD: 8 cinnamon rolls

1 tablespoon yeast
3 tablespoons warm water
1 cup sorghum flour
¼ cup cornstarch
¼ cup tapioca flour
1 tablespoon xanthan gum
4 tablespoons vegetable oil
3 tablespoons honey
½ cup soy milk
¼ teaspoon salt
1 egg
¼ cup butter (½ stick)
¼ cup sugar
1 tablespoon cinnamon
½ cup sorghum flour (reserve for kneading)
¼ cup finely chopped walnuts (optional)
¼ cup raisins (optional)

1. In a large bowl, dissolve the yeast in the warm water. Test the temperature of the water on the inside of your wrist—it should feel neither hot nor cold; you should not be able to feel it at all.
2. In a medium bowl, stir the sorghum flour, cornstarch, tapioca flour, and xanthan gum together. Mix well to get out any clumps.
3. In a small bowl, combine the oil, honey, and soy milk. Stir this mixture into the yeast. Then add the salt and the egg to the yeast mixture.
4. Gradually add the flour mixture to the yeast mixture. Once everything is mixed, stir vigorously for about 10 seconds. Cover the bowl with a dish towel and set in a warm place to rise for ½ hour.
5. Meanwhile, prepare the filling. Stir together the butter and sugar, then add the cinnamon. Set aside.
6. Once the dough has risen (it doesn't rise dramatically at this point), use some sorghum flour to liberally dust a countertop or cutting board, your hands, and the dough itself.

7. Knead the dough several times on the floured surface. Keep dusting with the extra flour if the dough becomes sticky.

8. Once the dough becomes handleable, form it into ropes, about 1 inch wide and 10 inches long.

9. Spread the butter mixture on one side of each rope. Sprinkle with chopped walnuts and stud with raisins if you choose to use them.

10. Starting at one end, roll up each rope to make cinnamon spirals. Place them on a greased cookie sheet, cover with a dish towel, and put them back in the warm place to rise for 1 hour.

11. Preheat the oven to 375°F and bake for about 15 minutes, until golden and gooey.

HINT

For fresh, warm cinnamon rolls in the morning, make the dough at night. Shape the rolls, and cover each roll with plastic wrap (but don't wrap them up). Instead of leaving them out for the second rise, put them in the fridge. The cool temperature will slow down the rising action, and they will be ready by morning. When you wake up, just pop them in the oven.

Polenta Breakfast Pudding

Creamy, hearty, and comforting . . . this thick hot cereal is simply delicious and will warm you on even the coldest winter morning.

PREP: 1 minute	¼ cup cornmeal
COOKING: 5 minutes	⅛ teaspoon salt
TOTAL TIME: 6 minutes	½ tablespoon butter
YIELD: 1 cup	1 tablespoon maple syrup
	¼ cup water
	¾ cup almond milk

1. Put all the ingredients in a pot on the stove over high heat.
2. Stir it constantly. Once it begins to bubble, cook for 1 minute longer, while continuing to stir.
3. Remove from the heat and spoon into a bowl . . . or enjoy straight from the pot.

To Serve Four:
1 cup cornmeal
½ teaspoon salt
2 tablespoons butter
3 tablespoons maple syrup
1 cup water
3 cups almond milk

Prepare as in previous steps and everyone will enjoy.

Easiest Eggs

Forget about omelets and scrambled eggs; they just create a big mess. This is the easiest and most delicious way to cook an egg. Minimal mess, minimal cleanup, and you don't need to hover over them while they cook. You will need small ceramic dishes, one for each serving. Ramekins are ideal: ceramic dishes that are roughly 3 inches in diameter with walls about 1 inch high. I use small, shallow heart-shaped dishes that are about as cute as you can get; you end up with heart-shaped eggs.

PREP: 1 minute

COOKING: 7 minutes

TOTAL TIME: 8 minutes

YIELD: 1 serving

¼ teaspoon olive oil
1 to 2 cups water
1 to 2 eggs
Dash salt
Dash pepper

1. Lightly coat the bottom and the sides of a ramekin with a dab of olive oil, cooking spray, or butter. Put the ramekin in a frying pan and place on the stove over high heat.
2. Pour water into the frying pan around the ramekin, so the water level is about one-third of the way up the side of the dish.
3. Crack one or two eggs into the ramekin. You can use just the egg whites for less fat: Two egg whites equal one egg.
4. Sprinkle with salt and pepper, and cover the pan with the lid slightly askew. The water will start to boil and cause the ramekin to clatter a little; this is normal. In 5 to 7 minutes you will have delicious and tender eggs.
5. Carefully lift the ramekin from the frying pan with a spatula or a pot holder, and slide the egg out with a fork.

HINT

- Before the egg starts to cook, season it with spices. Sprinkle on some dill or dried rosemary. As it cooks, the herbs infuse the whole egg with flavor.
- If there is too much water in the pan surrounding the ramekin, the water will "jump" over the walls of the ramekin when it boils and cause the egg to get wet. This is not a disaster, and cooking the egg for a bit longer with the lid off, at the end, will dry it up.

The Perfect Hard-Boiled Egg

Hard-boiling an egg is a great mystery—how do you know when they are done? Cooking for too long will turn the eggs to rubber, and cutting it short can be unappetizing. Here is the best and the easiest way to perfectly hard-boil an egg.

PREP: None

COOKING: 15 minutes

TOTAL TIME: 20 minutes

YIELD: 1 serving

1 egg
3 cups water

1. Put the egg in a pot. Note that you can cook as many eggs as you like, so long as they form a single layer in the pot.
2. Add enough water to cover the egg by 1 inch. Bring to a boil over high heat. Immediately remove the pot from the stove, cover, and let it sit for 10 minutes. Set a timer.
3. After 10 minutes, transfer the egg (gently) to a bowl of ice-cold water. This is important; otherwise, the egg would continue to cook itself. Let the egg sit in the cold water for 5 minutes.

HINT

You can store hard-boiled eggs in the fridge for up to one week. Hard-boiled eggs are easy snacks, great travel food, or a tasty addition to a green salad.

SMOOTHIES

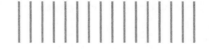

Smoothies are the ultimate quick meal. I've invented one for every mood, ranging from creamy fruit concoctions, to energizing vegetable smoothies, to rich and decadent treats. Each one is easy, healthy, and delicious.

SUPPLEMENTS AND ADDITIONS

Boost the nutritional value of a smoothie by adding any or all of the following supplements:

Flaxseed oil: Flaxseed oil is a rich source of essential fatty acids, of which 90 percent of Americans are deficient. The health benefits of flaxseeds are innumerable. Buy flaxseed oil in small amounts and store in the fridge. Flaxseed oil will make your smoothie thicker and creamier. Use 1 tablespoon per smoothie.

Flaxseed meal: Flaxseed meal is merely ground flaxseeds. Flaxseed meal provides the same nutritional benefits as flaxseed oil, along with fiber from the hulls. Use about 1 tablespoon per smoothie.

Spirulina: Spirulina is dried algae. It is an extremely dense form of protein, vitamins, and minerals. It's considered a "superfood." Spirulina has a distinct flavor that you soon get used to. Use 1 teaspoon per smoothie.

Protein powder: Protein powder can be made from soy, rice, eggs, or whey. Be aware that whey is derived from dairy, and be sure to choose a protein powder with no added gluten. Protein, combined with the complex carbohydrates found in fruits, can keep insulin levels steady and therefore provide more sustained levels of energy.

Common-Sense Disclaimer: I encourage you to research any vitamin or mineral supplements you feel may be helpful to your health and healing, and to discuss your options with knowledgeable nutritionists or medical professionals that you trust. Quality control is nebulous in the world of supplements, and educating yourself is important in order to choose the products that are right for you.

The Standard Smoothie

Simple and delicious—this is the smoothie from whence all smoothies came.

PREP: 3 minutes
COOKING TIME: None
TOTAL TIME: 3 minutes
YIELD: 2 cups

1 cup plain yogurt
1 cup frozen strawberries
1 squeeze of honey

1. Put all the ingredients into a blender.
2. Mix until smooth and sweet.

MAKE YOUR OWN FROZEN FRUIT

It's so easy. When particular fruits are in season, they become very inexpensive. Stock up on fresh fruit and store this fruit in the freezer. To freeze fruit for use in smoothies, wash the fruit and dry it completely, cut into small pieces, and put in freezer bags. Arrange the cut fruit in a flat layer in the bags, and freeze in this manner to keep the fruit from freezing into one giant clump.

Tropical Twist Smoothie

Fruits that are packed with enzymes combine with a hit of cayenne to aid digestion and help your body de-stress.

PREP: 5 minutes

COOKING: None

TOTAL TIME: 5 minutes

YIELD: 1½ cups

1 cup pineapple
1 tablespoon water or pineapple juice
1 cup papaya
½ lime
1 teaspoon agave nectar
⅛ teaspoon cayenne

1. Blend the pineapple along with a tablespoon of water or pineapple juice to help it mix.
2. Add the papaya, cayenne, and juice from half a lime, and then sweeten with agave nectar.
3. Blend well and be well.

HINT

Fresh pineapple and papaya each contain a powerful digestive enzyme. These are beneficial to everyone, especially people whose digestive systems are on the mend. Pineapple and papaya that have been canned, processed, cooked, or commercially frozen no longer contain these enzymes, as they are destroyed by high heat.

Sweet Shake

The taste is so decadent, yet the ingredients are so good for you. This power-packed smoothie provides energy and nutrition to get you through any day.

PREP: 5 minutes

COOKING: None

TOTAL TIME: 5 minutes

YIELD: 2 cups

1 cup plain soy milk
1 banana
1 heaping tablespoon almond butter
½ cup frozen raspberries

1. Blend the soy milk, banana, and almond butter until creamy and smooth.
2. Add the raspberries and blend again. So divine.

Punch It Up

This smoothie is like a glass of sunshine just for you, bursting with fresh fruit, fabulous flavors, and vitamins to rev up your body.

PREP: 5 minutes

COOKING: None

TOTAL TIME: 5 minutes

YIELD: 2½ cups

1 pink grapefruit
1 orange
1 banana
6 strawberries

1. Cut the grapefruit in half and squeeze all the juice into the blender.
2. Add the orange and banana and blend.
3. Add the strawberries and blend again. Pow!

HINT

Wait to wash fresh berries until right before you use them. Washing them in advance will cause them to get kind of soggy and they go bad quickly.

Creamy Dream Smoothie

One taste of this creamy shake will take you to cloud nine. Mild, rich almond butter tastes divine with the bright sweetness of a fresh, ripe peach.

PREP: 3 minutes

COOKING: None

TOTAL TIME: 3 minutes

YIELD: 1½ cups

1 cup plain soy milk
2 tablespoons almond butter
1 fresh peach

1. Blend the soy milk and almond butter until creamy and smooth.
2. Add the peach and blend again. Enjoy.

Mock Mimosas

This smoothie is bright and tingly and will give you a buzz of energy.

PREP: 3 minutes

COOKING: None

TOTAL TIME: 3 minutes

YIELD: 2 cups

1 orange
2 apricots
Juice of 1 lime

1. Peel the orange and blend with the apricots.
2. Squeeze the lime juice into the blender. Blend again and enjoy.

THE BENEFITS OF RAW FOOD

Fresh, raw fruits and veggies contain enzymes that work with the digestive system and help maintain the body's own store of enzymes. Over time, eating plenty of raw foods every day has a restorative effect on the body's digestive capacities.

V-8000

Your body will love you.

PREP: 7 minutes
COOKING: None
TOTAL TIME: 7 minutes
YIELD: 2 cups

½ of a cucumber
3 Roma tomatoes or 1 beefsteak tomato
½ of a green bell pepper
⅛ cup water
5 large spinach leaves
4 sprigs of flat-leaf parsley
1 small garlic clove or ½ large clove
Dash hot sauce
Dash sea salt

1. Peel the cucumber. Chop the cucumber, tomatoes, and bell pepper into large pieces and blend with the water.
2. Add the spinach and parsley leaves.
3. Press the garlic clove and add it to the blender along with a few shakes of hot sauce and a dash of sea salt.
4. Blend well and enjoy immediately.

Blue Banana Smoothie

This smoothie is not only healthy but healing as well. Blueberries, bananas, and the spices used are known to soothe and treat a distressed stomach.

PREP: 5 minutes	1 cup plain soy milk
COOKING: None	½ banana
TOTAL TIME: 5 minutes	¾ cup frozen blueberries
YIELD: 2 cups	½ teaspoon ground cinnamon
	¼ teaspoon ground ginger
	Dash nutmeg
	1 tablespoon honey

1. Blend the soy milk, banana, and blueberries until creamy.

2. Add the spices and honey and blend again. Enjoy.

HINT

Measurements do not need to be exact. Altering recipes around your particular tastes is part of the wonderful freedom that comes with preparing your own food. For a milder smoothie, cut the honey and add more banana.

Desert Dessert

Dates are crystallized sunlight, rich and sweet. For those who can no longer enjoy chocolate because of a milk intolerance, or for those who prefer a healthier alternative, this sweet, heavenly shake will knock out the fiercest cravings.

PREP: 5 minutes

COOKING: None

TOTAL TIME: 5 minutes

YIELD: 2 cups

1 cup plain soy milk
1 banana
4 large dates (about ⅓ cup)
¼ teaspoon nutmeg
2 teaspoons carob or cocoa powder
    (optional)

1. Blend the soy milk and banana, then add the dates and nutmeg and blend until frothy.
2. Add the carob or cocoa if you crave it. Mmmmmmmmmmmmm.

Power Punch

This is fantastic! The intense flavors of apple and pineapple dominate this gorgeous drink, packed with the nutrition of fresh spinach. You truly cannot taste the spinach at all.

PREP: 5 minutes

COOKING: None

TOTAL TIME: 5 minutes

YIELD: 2 cups

1 cup canned pineapple and juice
1 small apple
1 cup fresh spinach leaves

1. Cut the apple into chunks and tear the stems off the spinach leaves.
2. Put the pineapple into the blender, then the apple, and then the spinach leaves on top.
3. Blend well, so everything becomes a frothy and beautiful pale green delight.

Coconut Bliss

This exotic and delectable treat makes any day a vacation from normal. Delicious, nutritious, and very filling.

PREP: 10 minutes

COOKING: None

TOTAL TIME: 10 minutes

YIELD: 2½ cups

1 young coconut
½ mango
1 banana

1. Open the coconut as described on page 99.
2. Pour the coconut water into the blender. Scoop out the coconut meat and add that to the blender as well. Blend.
3. Peel the mango with a carrot peeler, and slice ½ of it into the blender.
4. Add the banana and blend into a lovely thick shake.

Peanultimate Smoothie

A rich, creamy shake loaded with nutrition.

PREP: 3 minutes

COOKING: None

TOTAL TIME: 3 minutes

YIELD: 1½ cups

1 cup plain soy milk
1 banana
2 heaping tablespoons peanut butter

1. Blend the soy milk and banana until creamy and smooth.

2. Add the peanut butter and blend again. Drink slowly and savor.

HINT

■ Use frozen banana for a thicker drink.

■ Add 1 teaspoon carob or cocoa powder if you crave it.

Super Deluxe Smoothie

This smoothie is liquid energy. You won't need coffee when you start your day with this powerful blend of fruits, essential fats, and valuable minerals.

PREP: 5 minutes

COOKING: None

TOTAL TIME: 5 minutes

YIELD: 1½ cups

1 orange
1 banana
1 tablespoon flaxseed oil
1 teaspoon agave nectar
1 teaspoon spirulina
6 large, fresh strawberries

1. Peel the orange, put into the blender with the banana, and blend.
2. Add the flaxseed oil, agave nectar, and spirulina, and blend again.
3. Add the strawberries and blend once more. Enjoy.

Green Tea Tonic

On those mornings when you make your tea and then forget about it, turn it into this fresh, light, energizing drink.

PREP: 3 minutes

COOKING: None

TOTAL TIME: 3 minutes

YIELD: 2 cups

1 cup cold green tea
3 apricots
1 teaspoon honey
½ cup ice

1. Blend the green tea and apricots; then add the honey while blending.
2. Add the ice and blend until crushed.

Heavenly Smoothie

Chocolate and raspberries are the ultimate combination. This thick, cold smoothie is dessert any time of day.

PREP: 3 minutes

COOKING: None

TOTAL TIME: 3 minutes

YIELD: 2 cups

1 cup chocolate soy milk
1 cup frozen raspberries
1 tablespoon flaxseed oil

1. Blend the soy milk and raspberries, then add the flaxseed oil while the blender is running.
2. Eat with a spoon . . . Mmmmmmmmmm.

HINT

Never cook with flaxseed oil. Heat destroys its beneficial properties and makes it taste bad. Buy flaxseed oil in small quantities and store it in the fridge to keep it fresh.

Papaya Pond Sludge

Papayas are rich in enzymes that aid in digestion and can relieve your system of stress. This thick drink allows your body to redirect energy toward healing or fighting off illness.

PREP: 5 minutes

COOKING: None

TOTAL TIME: 5 minutes

YIELD: 2½ cups

1 orange, or 1 cup orange juice
½ cup raspberries, or 1 peach
1 cup ripe papaya

1. Peel the orange and blend with the raspberries or peach until smooth.
2. Add the papaya, continue blending, and watch it thicken.
3. For true pond sludge and an extra boost of nutrition, add 1 teaspoon spirulina before adding the papaya.

Smooth Smoothie

Rich and delish, these dynamic flavors combine to create a cold thick smoothie that competes with the best strawberry ice cream.

PREP: 3 minutes

COOKING: None

TOTAL TIME: 3 minutes

YIELD: 2 cups

1 cup buttermilk
1 cup frozen strawberries
1 tablespoon maple syrup

1. Place all the ingredients in the blender.
2. Mix until smooth. Yum.

INVENT YOUR OWN SMOOTHIES

It's nearly impossible to make a bad smoothie. Putting different flavors together in unusual combinations can bring thrills to your palate.

Consider these tips for easy blending:

- Put liquids into the blender before you add solids.
- Soy milk blended with frozen fruit creates a thicker smoothie than achieved with other milks.
- Always add papaya last, after other ingredients have been blended. Papayas thicken up a smoothie to an alarming degree and can make further blending difficult.

Pumpkin Spice Smoothie

Pumpkin is not just for holidays. It's packed with vitamins, minerals, beta carotene, and fiber. Nourish your body with this cozy treat.

PREP: 5 minutes

COOKING: None

TOTAL TIME: 5 minutes

YIELD: 1½ cups

1 cup plain soy milk
½ teaspoon ground cinnamon
¼ teaspoon ground ginger
Dash ground nutmeg
Dash ground cloves
½ cup canned pumpkin
1 tablespoon maple syrup

1. Blend the soy milk and spices together.
2. Add the pumpkin and maple syrup, and blend until creamy.

TRIVIA

Cinnamon is the dried inner bark of a particular evergreen tree. It has been used medicinally for years.

Almond Milk

Almond milk is incredibly good but also incredibly time-consuming to make. It makes a lovely treat when you are really missing milk.

PREP: 10½ hours

COOKING: None

TOTAL TIME: 10½ hours

YIELD: 3 cups

1 cup raw almonds
Water

1. Cover the almonds with water and allow them to soak for 10 hours, or overnight. The almonds will plump up and almost double in size, so use a bowl or jar that is large enough to accommodate this.
2. Discard the soaking water. Put 1 cup of soaked almonds into the blender with 3 cups of fresh water, and blend on high speed until creamy. This can take a few minutes.
3. Line a sieve or funnel with two layers of cheesecloth. Pour the blended almonds into the sieve to strain.
4. Let it drain, then gather the ends of the cheesecloth and wring out the remaining liquid.
5. Put the pulp back into the blender, add 1½ cups of fresh water, and repeat the process.
6. This is almond milk! It will keep in the fridge for 3 days.

Tasty Variations
➤ For an absolutely divine Nut Nog, blend almond milk with a few dates and a dash of nutmeg.
➤ You can turn the strained pulp into almond flour. Spread it on a cookie sheet and put in a 250°F oven for several hours, until dry. You want to dehydrate it, not cook it. Once it is completely dry, grind it into flour in a blender or food processor.

HINT

Soaked almonds are a delicious treat by themselves. Peel them with your fingernail—this is easier to do when the almonds are wet. Nuts that have been soaked are easier to digest, and it is easier for the body to utilize the nutrients they contain. Store soaked almonds in the fridge in an airtight container for three to four days.

BREADS

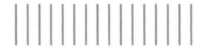

*Inevitably, once you learn you can never
eat bread again, it's all you crave.
Satisfy those cravings with the following recipes . . .
no one would ever know these breads are gluten free.*

BREAD TIPS

Flour Mixes

If there are any particular breads that you bake often, you can make the process speedier and easier by premixing the dry ingredients. Measure out the necessary flours, arrowroot, baking soda, baking powder, xanthan gum, and salt, and store each batch in individual ziplock bags. When you are ready to bake, just grab a bag—it's like using instant mix. Then add whatever other ingredients are necessary.

Baking Hints

Measuring honey can be sticky and difficult, but there's a simple trick. Coat the measuring cup or spoon with a touch of vegetable oil before using it to measure the honey. The honey will slide right out.

When cleaning flour off your countertop (or wherever it's spilled), use a dry towel to gather up as much of the flour as possible. Water combined with flour turns into glue and becomes an even bigger mess.

Buckwheat Banana Bread

A new version of a great classic, this hearty, flavorful bread has a fabulous cakelike texture.

PREP: 10 minutes

COOKING: 12 minutes for muffins
45 minutes for loaf

TOTAL TIME: 22 minutes for muffins
55 minutes for loaf

YIELD: 1 loaf or 12 muffins

4 very ripe bananas
⅓ cup vegetable oil
⅓ cup maple syrup
1 cup buckwheat flour
½ cup millet flour
2 tablespoons arrowroot
1 teaspoon baking powder
1 teaspoon baking soda
½ teaspoon xanthan gum
½ teaspoon salt
⅓ cup chopped walnuts

1. Preheat the oven to 325°F.
2. In a large bowl, mash the bananas with the oil and the maple syrup.
3. Mix all the other ingredients, except the walnuts, in another bowl.
4. Add the flour mix to the banana mixture and stir to combine. Then add the chopped walnuts.
5. Lightly grease a bread pan or a muffin pan with vegetable oil, and spoon the batter into the pan. If using a muffin pan, fill each muffin mold about three-quarters of the way.
6. Bake the bread loaf for 20 minutes, then remove from the oven and cover the loaf with a loose tent of tinfoil to prevent the top from getting burned. Bake for another 15 minutes or until a toothpick inserted into the center of the loaf comes out clean. Bake muffins for 12 minutes, and test for doneness with a toothpick as you would with the bread.

Almond Cakes

These delicate cakes don't use flour at all. Instead, they are made from almonds, which make them unique and satisfying.

Prep: 18 minutes

Cooking: 10 minutes

Total Time: 28 minutes

Yield: 12 muffins

1½ cups raw almonds
6 eggs whites
6 egg yolks
⅓ cup sugar
Juice of ½ orange (about ¼ cup)
¼ teaspoon orange zest
⅛ teaspoon ground cinnamon

1. Preheat the oven to 350°F.
2. Put the almonds into a dry blender and blend to create a flour. It should be fairly fine overall, with just a few larger almond bits.
3. Separate the eggs one by one. Beat the egg whites until they are stiff, and set aside.
4. In a large bowl, beat together the egg yolks and the sugar, then add the orange juice and zest and beat it well. Stir the cinnamon and almond flour into the egg yolk mixture.
5. Gently stir about 2 tablespoons of the egg whites into the egg yolk mixture, then very gently fold in the rest of the egg whites so that everything is mixed, but the egg whites are not crushed.
6. Grease a muffin pan and fill nearly to the top with batter.
7. Bake for 10 minutes and allow to cool, then remove cakes from tins and enjoy!

HINT

You can top these with whipped cream to turn them into a rich dessert.

Pumpkin Bread

Flavorful and rich, this is the perfect bread for brunch or tea or a midnight snack.

PREP: 15 minutes

COOKING: 45 minutes

TOTAL TIME: 1 hour

YIELD: 1 loaf

¾ cup pumpkin
1 egg
1 egg white
⅓ cup vegetable oil
1 cup sorghum flour
½ cup millet flour
¼ cup arrowroot
½ cup sugar
1 teaspoon baking powder
1 teaspoon baking soda
½ teaspoon xanthan gum
½ teaspoon salt
½ teaspoon ground cinnamon
¼ teaspoon ground ginger
¼ teaspoon ground nutmeg
¼ teaspoon ground cloves
¾ cup chopped walnuts

1. Preheat the oven to 325°F.
2. In a large bowl, mix the pumpkin, egg, egg white, and oil.
3. In another bowl, mix the flours and spices.
4. Stir the flour mix into the pumpkin mix, then add the chopped walnuts.
5. Thoroughly grease a bread pan with butter or vegetable oil. Pour the batter into the bread pan, and bake for 45 minutes.

HINT

Be sure to get plain canned pumpkin and not canned pumpkin pie mix, which is often on the same shelf.

Lace Crepes

These flavorful, savory crepes are fantastic hot from the frying pan. Teff has a rich nutty taste, and since it's a whole-grain flour, it is loaded with nutrition.

PREP: 3 minutes

COOKING: 2 minutes

TOTAL TIME: 5 minutes each

YIELD: 20 crepes

1 cup teff flour
½ teaspoon baking powder
2 cups soda water
2 tablespoons olive oil

1. Heat a frying pan over medium heat.
2. In a large bowl, mix the flour and baking powder together, and then add the soda water, which will be rather exciting. Whisk in the olive oil so the batter is smooth and thin.
3. Pour about ¼ cup of batter into the hot skillet. At the same time, make a swooping motion with the pan to allow the batter to spread out as thinly as possible in the pan. This creates wonderful unusual shapes with lacy patterns. To keep the crepe as thin as possible, don't use too much batter, and be sure to be swooping the frying pan with one hand as your pour it in.
4. Cook until tiny bubbles form, burst, and harden over the entire surface. The edges will begin to lift, and the whole thing will turn from light brown to dark brown. Don't flip it—it cooks on one side only, for about 2 minutes but up to 5 depending on how thick it is.

HINT

If you want to get creative, use a tablespoon to add the batter to the frying pan. You will need about 3 tablespoons' worth of batter, but this way you can make designs or spell things.

Cornbread

Moist and corny, this dense, crumbly bread is great for breakfast or perfect with soup.

PREP: 8 minutes

COOKING: 10 minutes

TOTAL TIME: 18 minutes

YIELD: 16 pieces

1 cup cornmeal
½ cup soy flour
1 teaspoon salt
1½ teaspoons baking powder
1 teaspoon baking soda
½ teaspoon xanthan gum
¾ cup soy milk
1 egg
¼ cup olive oil
¼ cup honey

1. Preheat the oven to 375°F.
2. Mix the dry ingredients in a large bowl. In another bowl, beat the soy milk, egg, and oil together, pour this over the dry ingredients, and stir to mix. Next, stir in the honey.
3. Lightly oil an 8-inch square baking dish or a large pie pan.
4. Pour the batter into the pan and bake for 10 minutes, or until a toothpick or knife inserted into the center of the cornbread comes out clean.

Puff Rolls

These soft, fluffy rolls are perfect for rainy, meditative days. They take time, and your home will smell wonderful.

PREP: 25 minutes

RISE: 1½ hours

COOKING: 15 minutes

TOTAL TIME: 2 hours, 10 minutes

YIELD: 12 rolls

1 tablespoon yeast
3 tablespoons warm water
1 cup sorghum flour
¼ cup cornstarch
¼ cup tapioca flour
1 tablespoon xanthan gum
4 tablespoons vegetable oil
3 tablespoons honey
½ cup soy milk
¼ teaspoon salt
1 egg
½ cup sorghum flour (reserve for kneading)

1. In a large bowl, dissolve the yeast in the warm water. Test the temperature of the water on the inside of your wrist—it should feel neither hot nor cold; you should not be able to feel it at all.
2. In a medium bowl, stir the sorghum flour, cornstarch, tapioca flour, and xanthan gum together. Mix well to get out any clumps.
3. In a small bowl, combine the oil, honey, and soy milk. Stir this mixture into the yeast.
4. Add the salt and the egg to the yeast mixture.
5. Gradually add the flour mixture to the yeast mixture. Once everything is mixed, stir vigorously for about 10 seconds. Cover the bowl with a dish towel, and set in a warm place to rise for ½ hour.
6. Once the dough has risen (it doesn't rise dramatically at this point), use some sorghum flour to liberally dust a countertop or cutting board, your hands, and the dough itself. Knead the dough several times on the floured surface. Keep dusting with the extra flour if the dough becomes sticky. Once the dough becomes handleable, form it into small, round rolls and place on a greased cookie sheet. Cover with a dish towel and put them back in the warm place to rise for 1 hour.
7. Preheat the oven to 375°F.

8. Bake for about 15 minutes, until the rolls are golden brown and hollow sounding when tapped on the bottom. Allow them to cool slightly before gobbling them up.

HINT

For shiny brown tops, brush the rolls with a beaten egg before baking.

Sopas

So cute! So easy! Sopas! These small corn cups are a lovely break from the norm. Fill with anything; fill with love.

PREP: 5 minutes

COOKING: 15 minutes

TOTAL TIME: 20 minutes

YIELD: 20 sopas

2½ cups corn flour
3 teaspoons baking powder
1 teaspoon sea salt
½ teaspoon ground cumin
1 cup soy milk
2 tablespoons oil

1. Preheat the oven to 350°F.
2. In a large bowl, mix the corn flour, baking powder, salt, and cumin. Add the soy milk and the oil, and stir everything together.
3. Take a piece of the dough and gently roll into a ball, roughly 1 inch in diameter. Indent the center of the ball and form it into a little cup with a flat bottom and raised edges. Repeat to use all the dough.
4. Place them on a lightly greased cookie sheet, and bake for 15 minutes.

Hot Crossbread

These fabulous mini-breads are a cross between a biscuit, a crumpet, and a pita. They make the perfect base for anything—honey and jam, a soft brie, hummus and tomato slices, or, of course, just plain.

PREP: 15 minutes

COOKING: 7 minutes

TOTAL TIME: 22 minutes

YIELD: 20

¾ cup soy flour
1 cup sorghum flour
1 teaspoon baking soda
2 teaspoons baking powder
½ teaspoon xanthan gum
¼ cup butter
⅓ cup soy milk
2 tablespoons honey

1. Preheat the oven to 350°F.
2. Mix the flours, baking soda, baking powder, and xanthan gum in a large bowl.
3. Add the butter with a fork or with your fingers so the mixture takes on a soft sandy texture. (It is far easier to use your fingers—and more fun.)
4. Gently stir in the milk and honey to form the dough.
5. Dust your hands with flour, take a piece of dough, and pat it between your hands to shape it into a round flat disk. It should be about 3 inches across and ¼-inch thin.
6. Place the disks on a greased baking sheet and bake for 6 to 8 minutes, until they slightly puff and turn golden brown.

HINT

- If you want to get ridiculously cute, roll the dough out on a floured surface to ¼-inch thick and cut out with cookie cutters.

- Make a double batch and toss half in ziplock bags in the freezer. Defrost in the toaster.

- These are great for road trips too.

Pizza Dough

End your pizza deprivation! There's no need to forego this favorite when you make your own crust.

<table>
<tr><td>

PREP: 25 minutes

RISE: 1½ hours

COOKING: 15 minutes

TOTAL TIME: 2 hours, 10 minutes

YIELD: 1 pizza

</td><td>

1 tablespoon yeast
3 tablespoons warm water
1 cup sorghum flour
¼ cup cornstarch
¼ cup tapioca flour
1 tablespoon xanthan gum
4 tablespoons vegetable oil
3 tablespoons honey
½ cup soy milk
¼ teaspoon salt
1 egg
½ cup sorghum flour (reserve for kneading)

</td></tr>
</table>

1. In a large bowl, dissolve the yeast in the warm water. Test the temperature of the water on the inside of your wrist—it should feel neither hot nor cold; you should not be able to feel it at all.
2. In a medium bowl, stir the sorghum flour, cornstarch, tapioca flour, and xanthan gum together. Mix well to get out any clumps.
3. In a small bowl, combine the oil, honey, and soy milk. Stir this mixture into the yeast. Then add the salt and the egg to the yeast mixture.
4. Gradually add the flour mixture to the yeast mixture. Once everything is mixed, stir vigorously for about 10 seconds, cover the bowl with a dish towel, and set in a warm place to rise for ½ hour.
5. Once the dough has risen (it doesn't rise dramatically at this point), use some sorghum flour to liberally dust a countertop or cutting board, your hands, and the dough itself.
6. Knead the dough several times on the floured surface. Keep dusting with the extra flour if the dough becomes sticky. Put the dough back in a bowl, cover it, and put it back in the warm place to rise for 1 hour.
7. Preheat the oven to 375°F.
8. Roll the dough into a large round pizza shape—if you don't have a rolling pin, use a bottle—and place it on a greased cookie sheet.

9. Cover your pizza with desired toppings (see page 150) and bake for about 15 minutes, until the crust is golden and the toppings are warm and bubbly.

HINT

Make more than one batch of dough, and freeze the extra. Shape the extra dough into a round crust directly on a cookie sheet lined with waxed paper. Put this in the freezer, as is. Once the dough has frozen, remove it from the cookie sheet and waxed paper, and wrap it tightly in plastic wrap. Perfect for spur-of-the-moment pizza cravings.

Rosemary Focaccia

Savory and crispy on the outside, tender and light inside, this large flatbread is quite wonderful.

PREP: 25 minutes

RISE: 1½ hours

COOKING: 15 minutes

TOTAL TIME: 2 hours, 10 minutes

YIELD: 9-inch focaccia

1 tablespoon yeast
3 tablespoons warm water
1 cup sorghum flour
¼ cup cornstarch
¼ cup tapioca flour
1 tablespoon xanthan gum
4 tablespoons vegetable oil
3 tablespoons honey
½ cup soy milk
¼ teaspoon salt
1 egg
1 tablespoon olive oil
1 tablespoon sea salt
1 tablespoon rosemary, crushed
½ cup sorghum flour (used for kneading and dusting)

1. In a large bowl, dissolve the yeast in the warm water. Test the temperature of the water on the inside of your wrist—it should feel neither hot nor cold; you should not be able to feel it at all.
2. In a medium bowl, stir the sorghum flour, cornstarch, tapioca flour, and xanthan gum together. Mix well to get out any clumps.
3. In a small bowl, combine the oil, honey, and soy milk. Stir this mixture into the yeast. Then add the salt and the egg to the yeast mixture.
4. Gradually add the flour mixture to the yeast mixture. Once everything is mixed, stir vigorously for about 10 seconds. Cover the bowl with a dish towel and set in a warm place to rise for ½ hour.
5. Once the dough has risen (it doesn't rise dramatically at this point), use some sorghum flour to liberally dust a countertop or cutting board, your hands, and the dough itself.
6. Knead the dough several times on the floured surface. Keep dusting with the extra flour if the dough becomes sticky.
7. Once the dough becomes handleable, form it into a flat puffy round and place on a greased cookie sheet or pie pan. Cover the dough again and put it back in the warm place to rise for 1 hour.

8. Preheat the oven to 375°F.

9. Liberally brush the top of the focaccia with olive oil, and sprinkle with coarse sea salt and crushed rosemary. You may use other herbs if you like.

10. Bake for about 15 minutes, until the top is a rich golden brown. Tap the bottom of the loaf with your fingernail; it should sound hollow when the bread is done.

11. Allow to cool slightly before cutting into wedges.

Wheatish Bread

A hearty roll that's reminiscent of whole wheat bread. Good for sandwiches.

PREP: 25 minutes

RISE: 1½ hours

COOKING: 15 minutes

TOTAL TIME: 2 hours, 10 minutes

YIELD: 8 rolls

1 tablespoon yeast
3 tablespoons warm water
½ cup sorghum flour
½ cup corn flour
¼ cup cornstarch
¼ cup tapioca flour
1 tablespoon xanthan gum
4 tablespoons vegetable oil
3 tablespoons honey
½ cup soy milk
—ONE → ¼ teaspoon salt
1 egg
½ cup sorghum flour (used for kneading and dusting)

1. In a large bowl, dissolve the yeast in the warm water. Test the temperature of the water on the inside of your wrist—it should feel neither hot nor cold; you should not be able to feel it at all.
2. In a medium bowl, stir the sorghum flour, corn flour, cornstarch, tapioca flour, and xanthan gum together. Mix well to get out any clumps.
3. In a small bowl, combine the oil, honey, and soy milk. Stir this mixture into the yeast. Then add the salt and the egg to the yeast mixture.
4. Gradually add the flour mixture to the yeast mixture. Once everything is mixed, stir vigorously for about 10 seconds. Cover the bowl with a dish towel and set in a warm place to rise for ½ hour.
5. Once the dough has risen (it doesn't rise dramatically at this point), use some sorghum flour to liberally dust a countertop or cutting board, your hands, and the dough itself.
6. Knead the dough several times on the floured surface. Keep dusting with the extra flour if the dough becomes sticky.
7. Once the dough becomes handleable, form it into patties and place on a greased cookie sheet. Cover with a dish towel and put them back in the warm place to rise for 1 hour.
8. Preheat the oven to 375°F.
9. Bake for about 15 minutes, until they are golden brown and hollow sounding when tapped on the bottom. Allow to cool slightly before using.

SOUPS

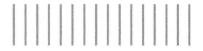

When I first began to cook, I began with soups.
Soups are wonderful: They are inexpensive,
easy to make, and are a full nutritious meal.
Devote an afternoon to making soup,
and you'll enjoy it all week long.

HOW TO STORE SOUP

Soup will keep in the fridge for about five days. Soups also freeze well, and last for two to three months in the freezer. To freeze soup properly, first cool it completely in the fridge. Overnight is best to ensure that it is cold throughout. Pour the soup into containers, no larger than 1 quart each. This is so the soup will freeze rapidly and prevent ice crystals from forming in the soup. *Do not* fill the containers all the way: Liquid expands as it freezes. When you're ready for the frozen soup, allow it to thaw, then reheat on the stove or in the microwave.

Chicken Vegetable Soup

This was the first soup I ever made, and I think it was all I ate for about three months. It's a two-day job, but worth it, and then you have soup for ages and it is wonderful.

PREP: 45 minutes

COOKING: Day 1: 3 hours
                   Day 2: 45 minutes

TOTAL TIME: 4½ hours over 2 days

YIELD: 20 cups

1 whole roasted chicken
1 yellow onion
10 carrots
5 leafy tops from celery stalks
About 15 cups water
7 celery stalks

1. Pull all of the meat off the roast chicken and set it aside. Put the skin and the carcass (all the bones) into a large stockpot.
2. Cut the onion into quarters and put two of the quarters into the pot. Wash three carrots but do not peel them. Break them in half and put them in the pot. Cut the leafy parts from the top of five celery stalks and put the leafy part into the pot.
3. Fill the pot with enough water to cover everything (about 15 cups). Bring to a boil, then turn down the heat so that it simmers gently. Cover with a lid that is slightly askew to allow some steam to escape. Simmer for about 3 hours.
4. Chop the chicken meat, the remaining half of onion, the celery stalks, and the remaining carrots into bite-size chunks, and put into a covered bowl in the fridge—you will not add these to the soup until day 2.
5. Once the broth has simmered for about 3 hours, strain the liquid into a large bowl (or multiple bowls) using a pasta strainer or colander. Throw away the chicken carcass and the vegetables; these were used to flavor the water and turn it into broth. Put the broth in the fridge overnight.
6. Overnight, the fat will rise to the top of the broth and harden. The next day, use a spoon to skim this layer of fat from the broth.
7. Put the broth back into the large soup pot and add the chicken meat and chopped vegetables. Bring to a boil, then turn down the heat and simmer for about 45 minutes.

HINT

For heartier soup, add to the broth six yellow potatoes, chopped into large chunks, with the chicken and other vegetables.

Potato Leek Soup

The subtle flavors of creamy potato and mild leek combine in this warm and wonderful soup.

PREP: 5 minutes

COOKING: 25 minutes

TOTAL TIME: 30 minutes

YIELD: 6 cups

1 tablespoon olive oil
1 yellow onion
2 cloves garlic
1 large leek
4 cups (1⅓ pounds) red potatoes
6 cups vegetable broth
¼ teaspoon black pepper

1. Heat the olive oil in a saucepan over medium heat.
2. Finely chop the onion and garlic, and sauté for a few minutes.
3. Cut the leek into thin slices, from the base to about halfway up the leaves. Chop the potatoes into small pieces.
4. Once the onions have sautéed, add the potatoes, leek, broth, and pepper to the saucepan.
5. Bring to a boil, then simmer, covered, for 15 minutes.
6. Mash up the potatoes a bit with a fork or by slicing through with a knife before serving.

HINT

Store onions away from potatoes and garlic; the onions will cause them to sprout.

Creamy Broccoli Soup

This soup is absolutely divine, incredibly beautiful, rich, delicious, comforting, and fabulous. Try it and see.

PREP: 15 minutes

COOKING: 20 minutes

TOTAL TIME: 35 minutes

YIELD: 4 cups

1 tablespoon olive oil
½ yellow onion
1 cup vegetable broth
4 cups (1 pound) broccoli florets
2 cups plain soy milk
½ teaspoon sea salt
¼ teaspoon black pepper

1. Heat the olive oil in a large saucepan.
2. Chop the onion and sauté for about 5 minutes. Add the broth and the broccoli florets, cover, and simmer for about 10 minutes, until the broccoli is quite tender.
3. Remove the saucepan from heat. Put the broccoli, onions, and broth into a blender and blend until quite smooth. Do not attempt to blend it all at once, rather, do it in two batches and use caution when blending hot ingredients.
4. Pour the creamy broccoli mixture back into the saucepan. Put the soy milk in the blender and blend for a moment, to mix with the residual broccoli puree, and pour into the saucepan.
5. Warm over medium heat, stirring often. Season with the salt and pepper to taste, and enjoy.

Carrot Soup

Creamy, warm, and slightly sweet, this is a surprisingly delicate and lovely soup.

PREP: 10 minutes

COOKING: 10 minutes

TOTAL TIME: 20 minutes

YIELD: 4½ cups

9 carrots
1 young coconut
½ teaspoon ginger
¼ teaspoon salt
Dash nutmeg

1. Peel the carrots and cut them into 2-inch chunks.
2. Steam the carrots until they become very tender and can be pierced easily with a fork.
3. Meanwhile, open the coconut (see page 99).
4. Put the coconut water, coconut meat, and spices into a blender and blend until frothy.
5. Once the carrots have steamed, add them one by one to the blender while it runs continuously. The heat of the carrots will warm the soup.

HOW TO OPEN A YOUNG COCONUT

Young coconuts, also called Thai coconuts or white coconuts, are different from the hard brown coconuts most people are familiar with. Young coconuts have a dense white husk surrounding them that looks like a little hut: It is cylindrical with a pointy top. The coconut is inside this husk. Young coconuts have lots of coconut water inside, which is more delicious than anything on earth and is extremely nutritious and pure. People can effectively perform blood transfusions using young coconut water if blood is not available—it has the same properties as blood plasma and assimilates into the body perfectly. The meat in young coconuts is a thin flexible layer that can be scraped out with a spoon. If these coconuts had aged further before harvesting, they would become old brown coconuts with tougher meat and less water inside.

Young coconuts are worth searching out because they are just incredible. You can find them in Asian and Latin American markets, and in some supermarkets or health food stores. I go to Chinatown in San Francisco for young coconuts, for they are often fresher and far less expensive than at health food stores.

Young coconuts are fabulous used in smoothies and in soup; however, drinking the water straight out of the coconut with a straw is beyond compare.

Choose coconuts that feel light. Heavy ones can be waterlogged and rotten. If you open the coconut and the water or meat has a lavender hue, it's bad and you have to throw it out. Fortunately, this is rare.

Opening young coconuts is easier than it would seem and makes a great party trick. You will need a sharp serrated bread knife, a strong pointy knife and hammer, and a large chef's knife.

1. With the serrated knife, saw off the husk from the pointy end.
2. You will see a small dome of coconut shell with three ridges that meet at the top and divide the dome into thirds. Two of the thirds will be the same size and one of the thirds will be slightly larger. Determine this.
3. You want to whack the coconut in the center of the largest third, about 1½ inches down from the top of the dome. Position the tip of the small pointy knife in this spot, and tap the handle with the hammer. You just want to get the blade through the shell.
4. If your chef's knife has a pointy butt-end where the blade meets the handle, you can aim and whack down with that to pierce the shell. I find this to be easier—just watch out for your hand.
5. Remove the knife and slide the point of the blade of the chef's knife into the slit you just made in the shell. Wiggle it in so that is firmly in the coconut. Then bring the knife handle straight up toward the ceiling—like prying the cap off a beer bottle. This motion will pop the top off the coconut in a perfect circle.
6. Enjoy . . . and prepare for your impending coconut addiction.

Hearty Beef Stew

As this soup simmers, your home will fill with a wonderful aroma. The flavors in the stew are even richer on the second day.

PREP: 45 minutes

COOKING: 1½ hours

TOTAL TIME: 2¼ hours

YIELD: 20 cups

2 yellow onions
6 carrots
5 cups (1 pound) button or cremini
   mushrooms
2 cups (¾ pound) green beans
2 pounds beef (see tip, page 101)
2 tablespoons olive oil
8 cups beef broth
4 cups chicken broth
2 bay leaves

1. Chop the onions, carrots, mushrooms, and green beans into large chunks. Cut the meat into 1-inch cubes.
2. Heat the oil in a large stockpot over a medium flame. Add the meat and lightly brown it on all sides. Add the onions and sauté for about 5 minutes.
3. Add the rest of the vegetables, the broth, and the bay leaves. Turn up the heat and bring to a boil.
4. Once the soup reaches a boil, turn the heat down so that the soup simmers gently. Cover with a lid that is slightly askew to allow steam to escape.
5. Simmer for about 1½ hours. It is now ready to eat.

Tasty Additions

For an even heartier stew, cut up and add four yellow potatoes. For more vitamin C, add a 28-ounce can of stewed tomatoes. If green beans are not in season, use celery instead, or use frozen green beans. If you use frozen beans, add them at the very end, in the last 15 minutes of cooking.

HINT

Bay leaves are used to flavor soups, but don't eat them. Remove them once the soup has cooked.

CHOOSING THE RIGHT STEW MEAT

Buy an inexpensive cut of meat such as a chuck roast, round steak, or pre-cubed stew meat. These cuts are not as tender as expensive steak, which is why they are cheaper. However, the long, slow cooking process of this stew will tenderize and flavor the meat to perfection.

Purely Vegetable Soup

Using nothing but pure water and the subtle flavors of vegetables, this is a gentle soup made from scratch. Enjoy this simple soup when you need to restart your system.

PREP: 10 minutes

COOKING: 2 hours

TOTAL TIME: 2½ hours

YIELD: 16 cups

1 leek
2 carrots
1 yellow onion
3 celery stalks with leafy tops
1 bay leaf
½ teaspoon peppercorns (or ground
    pepper)
16 cups cold water
sea salt, to taste

1. Trim the ends off the leek and cut into four large pieces. Wash the carrots but don't peel them. Cut off the ends and break them in half. Cut the onion into quarters, and cut the celery into thirds.
2. Put all the vegetables, the bay leaf, and the pepper into a large stockpot and cover with water.
3. Bring to a simmer over medium heat, then turn down to medium low. Cover, with the lid slightly askew, and simmer for 2 hours.
4. Strain the broth to trap the vegetables, peppercorns, and bay leaf, and throw them away.
5. Season the broth with sea salt and enjoy.

HINT

To build this broth into a wonderful veggie soup, you can add carrots, celery, green beans, tomatoes, potatoes, and squash to the broth. All you need to do is chop the chosen vegetables, add to the broth, and simmer for about 20 minutes.

Creamy Cauliflower Soup

You would swear this is a cream-based soup, but it's purely vegetable, which makes it very healthy and very filling.

PREP: 7 minutes

COOKING: 5 minutes

TOTAL TIME: 12 minutes

YIELD: 2 cups

4 cups cauliflower
1 cup water, or chicken or vegetable broth
2 tablespoons olive oil
½ teaspoon sea salt

1. Steam the cauliflower for about 3 minutes. It should pierce with a fork but still be firm.
2. Put the steamed cauliflower into a blender with the water or broth, olive oil, and salt. Blend until very smooth and creamy.
3. Warm it on the stove if necessary, and serve.

Tasty Addition

Sauté one clove of garlic and one thinly sliced shallot in 1 teaspoon of olive oil. Once sautéed, add 1 teaspoon of balsamic vinegar and sauté for 2 minutes more. Place a spoonful in the center of each cup of cauliflower soup. This is an elegant final touch and adds a burst of rich flavor.

Seafood Gumbo

Although a somewhat daunting recipe, this feast in a bowl is worth the effort. Thick and spicy, the flavors will blow you away.

PREP: 1 hour

COOKING: 2½ hours

TOTAL TIME: 3½ hours

YIELD: 24 cups

10 celery stalks
3 yellow onions
3 cloves garlic
3 tomatoes
1¼ pounds okra
½ cup flat-leaf parsley, minced
¾ cup vegetable oil
½ cup teff flour
½ cup arrowroot
8 cups vegetable broth
¼ cup Worcestershire sauce
4 bay leaves
2 teaspoons dried sage
2 teaspoons dried thyme
1 teaspoon dried oregano
1 teaspoon dried coriander
½ teaspoon cayenne
1 teaspoon black pepper
½ teaspoon sea salt
2 pounds shrimp (medium size, peeled, and deveined)
2 pounds white fish fillets (such as bass, halibut, or sole)

1. If your fish or prawns are frozen, take them out of the freezer to thaw.
2. Chop all the vegetables into small pieces. Put the celery, onion, and garlic into one bowl, the tomatoes into another bowl, and the okra and parsley into a third bowl.
3. In a large stockpot, combine the oil, the teff flour, and the arrowroot. Cook over medium heat for 20 minutes, stirring constantly. If you stop, it will burn. This is a long time! It goes faster if you sing.
4. After 20 minutes, add the celery, onion, and garlic. Cook for 5 minutes, stirring constantly.
5. Add the tomatoes and cook for 5 more minutes, stirring constantly.

6. Add the broth, Worcestershire, okra, parsley, and all the herbs and spices. Stir well to mix everything together. Put on a lid that is slightly askew so steam can escape, and bring to a simmer, still over medium heat.

7. Turn down the heat to the lowest possible setting while still maintaining a gentle simmer. Simmer, with the lid askew, for 1½ hours, stirring occasionally.

8. While it simmers, cut the fish into 1-inch pieces and peel and devein the shrimp.

9. After the soup has simmered for 1½ hours, add the fish and shrimp. Turn the heat back up to medium, and bring the soup up to a strong simmer. Remove the lid and simmer for 15 minutes, stirring occasionally.

10. Stir well and take a discerning taste. If it needs a bit more kick, slowly add cayenne and coriander, by the ¼ teaspoonful. Enjoy and be proud!

ABOUT THE SHRIMP

You can buy shrimp in many forms—peeled or unpeeled, raw or cooked. For this recipe, buy any kind you like. If they are unpeeled, you will need to peel and devein them. Take the tails off too. If you have the choice, buy fresh, raw shrimp, and the gumbo will cook them. Sometimes it is easier or cheaper to find frozen, precooked shrimp, and these work just fine too. Do be sure they are medium size, not small shrimpy shrimp.

Mushroom Tomato Soup

You will love curling up with a bowl of this creamy soup, popping with tomato flavor.

PREP: 5 minutes

COOKING: 15 minutes

TOTAL TIME: 20 minutes

YIELD: 6 cups

½ yellow onion

1 cup (⅓ pound) button or cremini mushrooms

3 tablespoons vegetable oil

3 tablespoons sorghum flour

1 clove garlic

4 cups vegetable broth

2 6-ounce cans tomato paste

1 cup plain soy milk

1 teaspoon dried basil

½ teaspoon sea salt

1. Dice the onion and slice the mushrooms.
2. Put the oil and flour in a saucepan over medium heat, and stir continuously for 5 minutes.
3. Add the garlic, onion, and mushrooms, and stir frequently. If it seems to be cooking too fast, add a little broth to the pan, about ¼ cup. Sauté for 5 minutes.
4. Add about 2 cups of the vegetable broth, then add the tomato paste. Stir until the paste becomes completely smooth.
5. Add the rest of the broth, the soy milk, basil, and the salt. Stir well, and heat through. Curl up and enjoy.

Miso Soup

This soup may sound unusual, but it is mild and delicious. It is quite filling and very easy to digest.

PREP: 5 minutes

COOKING: 10 minutes

TOTAL TIME: 15 minutes

YIELD: 6 cups

8 cups cold water

2 3-inch pieces of dulse seaweed

1 small leek

5 shitake mushrooms

1½ cups firm tofu

5 tablespoons red miso

12 spinach leaves

1. Put the water and the seaweed into a pot over medium-high heat. Heat the seaweed water for 7 minutes.
2. Meanwhile, thinly slice the leek and mushrooms, and cut the tofu into small cubes.
3. Remove the seaweed from the pot, and add the leek, mushrooms, and tofu to the broth. Heat for 3 minutes, then remove the pot from the heat.
4. Put the miso into a small bowl with a few spoonfuls of broth, and stir to dissolve it completely. Once dissolved, mix the miso into the soup.
5. Add the spinach leaves; they will wilt slightly from the heat of the broth. Enjoy.

HINT

While cooking this soup, it is important that the broth never reach a boil. It will steam and tiny bubbles form, but do not let it boil.

Tasty Variation

Using different seaweeds will impart a slightly different flavor to the broth. Experiment.

Lentil Soup

This soup is definitely a meal, perfect for autumn evenings or wintry days. You are in for some goodness.

PREP: 20 minutes

COOKING: 2½ hours

TOTAL TIME: 3 hours

YIELD: 12 cups

3 cups dried lentils
4 cups chicken or vegetable broth
3 cups cold water
2 cloves garlic
1 yellow onion
2 tomatoes
4 carrots
4 celery stalks
1 cup broccoli
½ teaspoon pepper
1 teaspoon dried oregano
1 tablespoon balsamic vinegar

1. Rinse the lentils and put them into a large stockpot with the broth and the water. Bring to a boil, then turn down to low heat and simmer, covered, for 1 hour.
2. In the meantime, mince the garlic and onions, and chop the vegetables into bite-size pieces.
3. Once the lentils have simmered for 1 hour, add the garlic, onion, tomatoes, and spices. Continue to simmer, covered, and over low heat, for another hour.
4. Add the carrots, celery, broccoli, and vinegar, and simmer for one last half hour. Now it's time to eat!

Gazpacho

Those who have had this fresh cold soup go crazy for it, even dream about it. Try it once and you'll be hooked.

PREP: 40 minutes

COOKING: None

TOTAL TIME: 40 minutes

YIELD: 16 cups

3 green bell peppers
2 red bell peppers
1 cucumber
1 jalapeño
6 large tomatoes
¼ cup cold water
2 tablespoons red wine vinegar
2 tablespoons olive oil
2 cloves garlic
1½ teaspoon sea salt
Dash hot sauce
Fresh cilantro (optional)

1. Dice the bell peppers and put them into a very large bowl. Cut the cucumber into quarters lengthwise; slice out the center seeded part; and throw it away. Chop up the cucumber and add it to the bowl.
2. Cut two tomatoes into quarters and put them into a blender. Slice the jalapeño in half and remove the seeds. Add the jalapeño to the blender, along with the water, vinegar, olive oil, garlic cloves, and salt. Blend well until completely smooth.
3. Cut the other tomatoes into quarters, add to the blender, and blend until smooth. You may need to blend the remaining tomatoes in two batches—use some of the puree to make it easier.
4. Pour the tomato puree into the large bowl with the cucumber and bell peppers and stir all this beauty together.
5. Shake in some hot sauce if desired, and top with fresh cilantro if you want to get fancy.

HINT

- Store tomatoes at room temperature. They lose flavor when you put them in the fridge.
- Make this soup with produce from your local farmers' market . . . it will taste even better.

SALADS
AND SIDES

||||||||||||||||||

*These simple and creative side dishes
are diverse enough to fend off boredom.
Use a single recipe to prepare a nutritious snack
or to complement a dinner, or combine
multiple recipes from this section to create
a fun multicourse meal.*

Salad Tepoz

Stunning flavors and textures combine to create this refreshing yet filling salad. Because of the avocado, there is no need for a dressing on this salad. The flavors are amazing on their own.

PREP: 15 minutes

COOKING: None

TOTAL TIME: 15 minutes

YIELD: 10 cups

1 head romaine lettuce
1 avocado
1 ripe pear
5 celery stalks
Handful of alfalfa sprouts
1 teaspoon sea salt
¼ to ½ teaspoon ground cumin

1. Tear the lettuce into a very large bowl.
2. Cut the avocado, pear, and celery into pieces, and add to the lettuce. Throw in the sprouts, and toss everything together.
3. Sprinkle a generous amount of sea salt over the salad, dust with ground cumin, and toss.
4. Let the salad sit for 5 minutes, then eat!

HINT

Don't be afraid of salt. Natural sea salt is essential to maintaining a healthy body. It has an incredible flavor and is a source of trace minerals, and it helps bring out the flavors of other foods.

Italian Greens

Fresh herbs add special dimension to this pungent and flavorful salad.

PREP: 15 minutes

COOKING: None

TOTAL TIME: 15 minutes

YIELD: 8 cups

1 head romaine lettuce
½ cup fresh basil
½ cup flat-leaf parsley
2 tomatoes
1 green bell pepper
4 hard-boiled eggs (optional, but highly recommended)
Sea salt
Black pepper

1. Tear the lettuce into a bowl. Chop the basil and parsley, or tear into small bits.
2. Chop the tomatoes, bell pepper, and eggs, and toss everything together.
3. Season with generous amounts of sea salt and black pepper. The flavors are best appreciated when only a simple olive oil is used as dressing.

HINT

To keep salad greens fresh for as long as possible, wash them in cold water and dry completely, then store in a Ziplock plastic bag with a paper towel.

Sunshine Salad

A divine combination of elegant flavors, bursting with sweetness and goodness.

PREP: 7 minutes	1 orange
COOKING: None	1 pink grapefruit
TOTAL TIME: 7 minutes	1 cup pineapple
YIELD: 3 cups	2 tablespoons Basic Balsamic Vinaigrette (page 176)

1. Peel the orange and cut the segments in half.
2. Peel the grapefruit and remove the membrane from around each individual segment.
3. Cut the pineapple into chunks.
4. Toss the fruit together in a bowl and drizzle with the balsamic dressing. So good!

Strawberry Spinach Salad

Elegant and easy, this is a delicious way to eat your spinach.

PREP: 15 minutes

COOKING: None

TOTAL TIME: 15 minutes

YIELD: 6 cups

6 cups fresh spinach (about ¾ bunch)
1 pint fresh strawberries (about 15 berries)
Basic Balsamic Vinaigrette (page 176), to
    taste
2 ounces goat cheese

1. Wash the spinach and tear off the stems. Dry well and tear into a bowl.
2. Slice the strawberries and toss them with the spinach.
3. Drizzle with Basic Balsamic Vinaigrette and toss to coat the spinach.
4. Crumble the goat cheese over the top of the salad.

Sexy Salad

This is my favorite. Try this incredible combination of flavors and textures and I'll wager it will become your favorite too.

PREP: 10 minutes

COOKING: None

TOTAL TIME: 10 minutes

YIELD: 6 cups

½ head green leaf lettuce
1 mango
1 avocado

1. Tear the lettuce into small bits.
2. Peel and cut the mango and avocado into chunks.
3. Toss the lettuce, avocado, and mango together in a large bowl.
4. Don't use dressing on this salad. It really doesn't need any. The avocado and mango do something wonderful together . . .

HINT

Peeling a mango is easy with a carrot peeler. Peel off the rind (sometimes you need to go over it twice), then slice the mango fruit from the center seed in big pieces and cut into chunks.

Summertime Salad

This unusual combination of crisp, delicious flavors will have you smiling uncontrollably. Fresh and festive, this salad is a huge hit.

PREP: 10 minutes

COOKING: None

TOTAL TIME: 10 minutes

YIELD: 7 cups

5 cups watermelon (about 3½ pounds)
1½ cups jicama (about ¼ pound)
1 cup celery (about 3 stalks)
½ jalapeño

1. Cut the watermelon into slices and use a paring knife to cut off the rind. Cut into bite-size pieces.
2. Cut the jicama into a few large pieces, and slice off the skin with a knife. Cut into small cubes.
3. Chop the celery.
4. De-seed the jalapeño and mince.
5. Put all these lovely things into a large bowl and mix them up.
6. Serve as is, or over a bed of romaine lettuce.

Exotic Steak Salad

This stunning steak salad is a feast for your eyes as well as your stomach. Beautiful colors and surprising flavors marry in this delicious, satisfying salad that won't leave you feeling heavy.

PREP: 10 minutes

COOKING: 15 minutes

TOTAL TIME: 20 minutes

YIELD: 8 cups

1 pound steak
¼ teaspoon sea salt
¼ teaspoon pepper
½ head romaine lettuce
2 cups papaya
1 yellow bell pepper
Sweet Rice Vinaigrette (page 177)

1. Dust each side of the steak with salt and pepper, and place it on a baking sheet lined with tinfoil. Move the oven rack to the topmost position, and set the oven to broil. Always leave the oven door slightly open while broiling. Broil the steak for 8 minutes, flip it over, and broil the other side for 6 minutes.
2. Meanwhile, tear the romaine, peel and cube the papaya, and chop the bell pepper.
3. Once the steak has cooked, let it sit for about 5 minutes before cutting into it. Slice the steak into thin slabs.
4. Create a nest of lettuce for the steak to lay upon, and artfully heap the papaya and bell pepper over the steak.
5. Drizzle with Sweet Rice Vinaigrette and enjoy.

Sweet Cukes

Delicate marinated cucumbers make a wonderfully cool and refreshing side dish or snack.

PREP: 5 minutes

COOKING: None

TOTAL TIME: 5 minutes

YIELD: 1½ cups

½ cup rice vinegar
1 cup water
¼ cup agave nectar
1 English cucumber

1. In a bowl, stir together the rice vinegar, water, and agave nectar.
2. Peel the cucumber and slice it into thin rounds, the thinner the better. I find using a cheese slicer makes this very easy.
3. Add the cucumber slices to the sweet vinegar bath like beautiful floating petals.
4. Refrigerate for 2 hours before eating. You can keep the cukes in the marinade for as long as you like.

Grilled Portobellos

These thrill me. They are great with steak or chicken, are a wonderful addition to salads, and are absolutely divine on their own.

PREP: 5 minutes

COOKING: 4 minutes

TOTAL TIME: 9 minutes

YIELD: 4 portobellos

4 portobello mushrooms
2 tablespoons balsamic vinegar
2 tablespoons olive oil
1 clove garlic
½ teaspoon sea salt
¼ teaspoon black pepper

1. Wipe off the mushrooms to clean them; don't wash them. Remove the stems.
2. Put the portobellos on a baking sheet with their undersides facing up.
3. In a small bowl, mix the vinegar, oil, garlic, salt, and pepper with a fork so it becomes thick and smooth. Spoon this over the mushrooms, reserving about one-third to use later.
4. Put the oven rack in the topmost position, and set the oven to broil.
5. Broil the portobellos for 3 minutes with the oven door slightly open.
6. Take them out and flip the mushrooms over. Spoon the remaining balsamic mixture over the tops and broil for 1 more minute.

Steamed Veggies

Steamed vegetables are quick, easy, filling, healthy, and loaded with nutrition and flavor. Add more veggies to your diet, and you will see an improvement in your skin and your vitality.

PREP: 2 minutes

COOKING: 10 minutes

TOTAL TIME: 12 minutes

YIELD: 2 cups

2 cups vegetables: try broccoli, zucchini, yellow squash, carrots, or cauliflower

1. Cut up the vegetables if necessary. All the pieces should be roughly the same size, but not too small or they risk getting mushy.
2. Bring 1 or 2 inches of water to a boil in a covered pot that fits a steamer basket.
3. Put the veggies in the steamer basket over the water and put the lid on the pot.
4. Steam anywhere from 3 to 10 minutes, depending on the vegetable and how tender you like it. Test by stabbing with a fork, and tasting it, of course.

Balsamic Sauté

Earthy flavors combine with a dynamic burst of balsamic in this easy dish. This sauté is fantastic with warm polenta or brown rice.

PREP: 5 minutes

COOKING: 7 minutes

TOTAL TIME: 12 minutes

YIELD: 4 cups

1 yellow onion
2 tomatoes
1 cup button or cremini mushrooms
½ head spinach
2 tablespoons olive oil
1 clove garlic
2 tablespoons balsamic vinegar

1. Chop the onion, tomatoes, and mushrooms, and tear the stems off the spinach leaves.
2. Heat the oil in a frying pan and sauté the garlic and onion.
3. Add the mushrooms, and after a few moments, the tomatoes.
4. Pour in the balsamic vinegar and add the spinach leaves.
5. Stir it up a bit and let it steam for about 3 minutes.

Roasted Roots

Hearty and tasty, the gorgeous combination of vibrant colors, fabulous aromas, and amazing flavors of these roasted vegetables will overcome your senses.

PREP: 10 minutes

COOKING: 35 minutes

TOTAL TIME: 45 minutes

YIELD: 6 cups

2 sweet potatoes
2 beets
2 carrots
1 parsnip
1 turnip
1 yellow onion
10 button or cremini mushrooms
3 tablespoons olive oil
½ teaspoon rosemary
½ teaspoon sea salt
Dash pepper

1. Preheat the oven to 375°F.
2. Peel all the vegetables. Roughly chop them into chunks, and cut the mushrooms in half if they are large.
3. Put the vegetables into a large baking dish and drizzle with olive oil. Sprinkle with rosemary, salt, and pepper, and gently toss so that everything gets coated.
4. Roast in the oven for 30 to 35 minutes, until tender. Stir them halfway through cooking if you think of it.

Steak Fries

These monster wedges will have you clamoring for more.

PREP: 5 minutes

COOKING: 30 minutes

TOTAL TIME: 35 minutes

YIELD: 12 fries

1 russet potato
1 yam or sweet potato
2 tablespoons olive oil
½ teaspoon sea salt

1. Preheat the oven to 350°F.
2. Cut the potatoes in half lengthwise, and then cut each half into thirds lengthwise, so that from each potato you get six long wedges.
3. Arrange the wedges on a cookie sheet, balanced on the curvy side of the potato (rather than resting on one of the flat sides).
4. Drizzle with olive oil and use your fingers to coat each wedge. Sprinkle with sea salt.
5. Bake for 30 minutes, and devour.

HINT

You can use as many potatoes as you like, depending on how many people you are serving.

Steamed Artichokes

Artichokes may look daunting, but they are actually quite easy to cook. They are such fun to eat, simultaneously elegant and frivolous, and have a great, unique flavor. Artichokes are delicious plain, though many people like to dip the leaves in butter, mayo, or olive oil.

PREP: 1 minute

COOKING: 40 minutes

TOTAL TIME: 40 minutes

YIELD: 2 artichokes

2 artichokes
15 cups water

1. Cut off the stems so the artichokes can sit flat. Put them in a stockpot and add enough water to cover the artichokes. Bring to a boil and boil for 30 to 45 minutes.
2. Test that they are done by pulling out a leaf. If it comes off easily, it is ready.
3. Drain the artichokes by setting them upside down for a moment.
4. They are delicious hot or cold.

HINT

Choose firm artichokes with tightly packed leaves.

Quinoa

This amazing food has been cultivated in South America since 3000 B.C. It is a high-quality complete protein, as it contains all eight essential amino acids. It is also high in iron and B vitamins. Quinoa is not a grain; it's related to beets, spinach, and chard.

PREP: 2 minutes

COOKING: 15 minutes

TOTAL TIME: 20 minutes

YIELD: 2 cups

1 cup quinoa
1½ cups water, or chicken or vegetable broth

1. Rinse the quinoa until the water runs clear.
2. Put the quinoa into a pot with the water or broth.
3. Bring to a boil, then turn down to low heat, cover, and simmer for 15 minutes.

HINT

Quinoa is as fast and as easy to cook as pasta. It lends itself well to the flavors of Spanish, Mexican, and Asian cuisine. Stir in fresh salsa to spice it up, or serve as a side dish with fish or chicken.

Millet

Millet is an ancient grain that humans have eaten since the Stone Age. It's a whole grain, and therefore highly nutritious and high in protein, as well as an excellent source of B vitamins and iron. Millet is considered the most easily digested grain available.

PREP: 2 minutes

COOKING: 30 minutes

TOTAL TIME: 35 minutes

YIELD: 2 cups

1 cup millet
2 cups water, or chicken or vegetable broth

1. Put the millet into a pot with the water or broth.
2. Bring to a boil, then turn down to low heat, cover, and simmer for 30 minutes. Once cooked, fluff with a fork.

HINT

Many flavors complement this healthy grain, so be creative. Serve as a side dish with meat or fish, or, once the millet has cooked, stir in any fresh vegetables you have on hand to create a beautiful pilaf.

Brown Rice

Brown rice is high in B vitamins, minerals, and insoluble fiber. White rice, however, has been milled and polished to remove the bran, which happens to be where most of the nutrition in rice is found.

PREP: 2 minutes

COOKING: 40 minutes

TOTAL TIME: 45 minutes

YIELD: 3 cups

1 cup brown rice

2 cups water, or chicken or vegetable broth

1 tablespoon olive oil (optional)

1. Rinse the rice until the water runs clear.
2. Put the rice into a pot with the water or broth, and the oil.
3. Bring to a boil, then turn down to low heat, cover, and simmer for 40 minutes. Resist lifting the lid until completely cooked.

HINT

■ Substitute brown rice for white rice whenever possible for greater nutritional bang for your buck. Since brown rice does take longer to cook, prepare a lot at once and keep the extra in the fridge for up to five days, to reheat in minutes.

■ Before cooking any rice, it is wise to rinse it until the water runs clear. Rice can be coated with talc, barley flour, or who knows what.

Lentils

Lentils have been around since 7000 B.C. These earthy legumes are high in calcium, iron, and B vitamins.

PREP: 2 minutes

COOKING: 30 minutes

TOTAL TIME: 35 minutes

YIELD: 2½ cups

1 cup dried lentils
2 cups water

1. Rinse the lentils and put into a pot with the water.
2. Bring to a boil, then turn down to low heat, cover, and simmer for 30 minutes. Do not add salt to the water, as it will make the lentils tough.

HINT

- Lentils are very inexpensive and make a filling side dish that goes well with steamed veggies or chicken.

- Experiment with seasonings. Once the lentils are cooked, try adding a touch of cumin and curry powder, or balsamic vinegar and thyme, or just simple sea salt and pepper.

Wild Rice

Wild rice is not truly rice, but the seed of a wild grass. Wild rice is chewy and fragrant, high in nutrients, with higher amounts of protein than white or brown rice.

PREP: 2 minutes

COOKING: 60 minutes

TOTAL TIME: 65 minutes

YIELD: 4 cups

1 cup wild rice
3 cups water

1. Briefly rinse the wild rice.
2. Put the rice into a pot with the water. Bring to a boil, then turn down the heat to low, cover, and simmer for 60 minutes.

HINT

Add some variety, and more nutrition, to your life with gorgeous wild rice. Try it in place of white rice in any of your favorite meals.

Hummus

A protein-rich dip for veggies and chips, hummus is a great mini-meal.

PREP: 15 minutes

COOKING: None

TOTAL TIME: 15 minutes

YIELD: 4 cups

¾ cup water
½ cup tahini
½ cup lemon juice
2 cloves garlic
2 teaspoons dill
1 teaspoon salt
⅛ teaspoon cayenne
3 cups canned garbanzo beans

1. Put the water, tahini, lemon juice, garlic, and spices into a blender and mix well.
2. Add the garbanzo beans in small batches of about a cup, and blend until thick and creamy. Repeat until all the beans are added.
3. Pour into a container and refrigerate to chill.

HINT

This recipe makes a lot! Keep some on hand in the fridge and freeze the rest.

Holy Guacamole

Few things are better than a giant bowl of fresh guacamole, and this, I have to say, is the absolute best. Be transported to fresh fantastic heaven.

PREP: 12 minutes

COOKING: None

TOTAL TIME: 12 minutes

YIELD: 6 cups

3 avocados
½ lime
1 jalapeño
2 green onions
2 small tomatoes
½ teaspoon cumin
1 teaspoon sea salt

1. Cut the avocados in half and use a spoon to scoop out the avocado into a big bowl.
2. Squeeze in the juice of half a lime, and mash the mixture with a fork. Leave it uneven and chunky.
3. Cut the jalapeño in half and cut out the seeds. The hotness of the jalapeño is in the pithy veins, so cut these out or leave them in depending on your taste. Without the pith and seeds, jalapeños are mild and have great flavor. Mince the jalapeño and toss into the guacamole.
4. Cut off and discard the top few inches of the green part of the green onions. Thinly slice the rest of the onion and add to the guacamole.
5. Cut the tomatoes into small pieces and add to the guacamole.
6. Sprinkle with cumin and salt, and mix everything together.

HINT

■ Put an avocado in a paper bag to speed its ripening.

■ Hot chilies stimulate endorphin production—the natural high. The hotter the chili, the more endorphins start flowing. Eat chilies and get happier.

■ Gone low carb? This guacamole is great spread onto a leaf of romaine, rolled up, and eaten like a little taco of deliciousness.

Power Pesto

Think Popeye. Toss with pasta, spread on chips, or eat by the spoonful; this pesto will have you zinging around with loads of energy.

PREP: 10 minutes

COOKING: None

TOTAL TIME: 10 minutes

YIELD: 1 cup

3 cups spinach
½ cup fresh basil
1 cup flat-leaf parsley
1 clove garlic
½ teaspoon sea salt
2 tablespoons olive oil

1. Wash the greens and tear off any thick stems.
2. Process the greens in a food processor with the S-blade, adding in one handful at a time.
3. Cut the garlic clove in half. Add the salt and one-half of the garlic to the greens.
4. Slowly pour in the olive oil while the food processor is running. Process to a smooth consistency, then taste.
5. If you would like more garlic, add the other half or one-half of the other half. Be careful; it gets strong fast.

HINT

- The measurements for the greens don't need to be precise—it's hard to mess up this recipe.

- To keep fresh basil lasting as long as possible, do not store it in the fridge. Instead, put the bunch of basil in a glass of water like a bouquet of flowers. It will easily last a week.

ENTRÉES

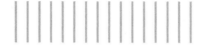

*A giant disadvantage of the gluten-free diet
is losing the convenience of ordering take-out
or nuking a frozen dinner. Bring back the ease
of "no-brainer" meals: Many of these dishes
take just moments to prepare, while others yield
plenty of leftovers to reheat at a moment's notice.*

"TAKE-OUT" FROM YOUR FREEZER

Bring back the ease and convenience of frozen dinners by making a variety of meals in advance. Devote part of a day to cooking a few different dishes. Package up the prepared food into individual servings—use small Tupperware containers, or wrap each serving in waxed paper and put them in a freezer bag. You will have a supply of delicious, easy meals to defrost whenever the mood strikes.

Baked Chicken

Ridiculously easy, and no dishes to wash, this is a very basic way to cook chicken in a hurry. Once the chicken is cooked, dip in BBQ sauce or hummus or to add to a salad or other entree. Dress up the chicken, if you like, by using a marinade. It's easy to cook as much or as little as you like.

1 to 4 chicken breasts

PREP: 1 minute

COOKING: 15 to 25 minutes

TOTAL TIME: 16 to 26 minutes

YIELD: 1 to 4 servings

1. Preheat the oven to 350°F.
2. Line a cookie sheet with tinfoil. Place the chicken on the cookie sheet, and bake for 15 to 25 minutes, depending on the thickness of the meat.
3. Test that the chicken is done by cutting into the meat: It should no longer be pink inside, and the juices should run clear.
4. Transfer the chicken to a plate, and enjoy with whatever side dishes you like.

Just Plain Chicken

This easy way to cook chicken breasts can be used in other recipes or in salads—no seasonings are used.

1 to 4 chicken breasts

PREP: None

COOKING: 10 to 15 minutes

TOTAL TIME: 15 minutes

YIELD: 1 to 4 servings

1. Put the chicken breasts into a pot and cover with water by 2 inches. Bring to a boil over high heat.
2. Boil, uncovered, for 10 to 15 minutes, depending on the thickness of the meat.
3. The chicken will turn white all the way through once it has cooked. Use this meat in salads or pasta dishes, or simply store in the fridge for when you need a quick bite—it's great cold, dipped in BBQ sauce.

Grilled Fish

In no time and with no hassle, you can prepare delicious grilled fish. Use this technique with any type of fish, with fillets or fish steaks.

PREP: 1 minute

COOKING: 8 minutes

TOTAL TIME: 9 minutes

YIELD: 1 serving

1 fish fillet or steak such as salmon,
   halibut, or sole
Dash pepper
Dash sea salt
1 tablespoon lemon juice

1. Set the oven to broil.
2. Line a cookie sheet with tinfoil and lightly coat it with oil.
3. Place the fish on the cookie sheet and season with pepper and sea salt. Squeeze a bit of lemon juice over the top if you have any, or try a dash of cayenne.
4. Broil for 8 minutes. Keep the oven door slightly open while broiling.
5. The fish is done when it turns opaque throughout and flakes easily.

HINT

Turn this dish into a stunning meal with Steamed Veggies (page 121), Roasted Roots (page 123), or the Italian Greens (page 113).

One Great Steak

The oven broiler is the unsung hero of the kitchen—it's like having an upside-down BBQ grill right in your oven. This is a simple, surefire way to cook a great steak—anyone can do it.

PREP: 1 minute

COOKING: 14 minutes

TOTAL TIME: 15 minutes

YIELD: 1 serving

1 steak (choose a nice thick steak, such as
    sirloin, rib eye, New York strip, or T-bone)
Pepper
Sea salt

1. Put the oven rack in its topmost position and set the oven to broil.
2. Season each side of the steak with pepper and sea salt. Place it on a cookie sheet lined with foil, with the edges pinched up to keep the juices from spilling over.
3. For a medium steak, broil for 8 minutes, flip the steak over, and broil for 6 minutes. For a rare steak, broil for 7 minutes, flip the steak over, and broil for 5 minutes. Keep the oven door partly open the entire time while broiling.
4. Take the steak from the oven and let it sit for a few minutes before you cut into it. This keeps it juicy and fabulous.
5. Turn off the broiler and keep the oven door open while it cools down.

HINT

Depending on your mood, some wonderful sides include the Strawberry Spinach Salad (page 115), Steak Fries (page 124), or Grilled Portobellos (page 120).

Inchilotta

Inspired by the delicious insides of an enchilada, this flavorful dish is fabulous hot or cold, as a salad or a casserole.

PREP: 15 minutes

COOKING: 30 minutes

TOTAL TIME: 45 minutes

YIELD: 8 cups

1 pound chicken breasts
½ cup lemon juice
1 teaspoon oil or cooking spray
¼ teaspoon sea salt
¼ teaspoon black pepper
Dash cayenne
1 sweet onion
2 tomatoes
2 15-ounce cans black beans
¾ teaspoon ground cumin
½ teaspoon dried sage
½ teaspoon sea salt
½ teaspoon black pepper
⅛ teaspoon cayenne
Corn tortilla (optional)

1. Preheat the oven to 350°F.
2. Put the chicken in a bowl with the lemon juice and let it sit in the fridge for 10 minutes.
3. Line a baking sheet with foil and lightly coat with oil or cooking spray.
4. Place the chicken on the baking sheet, sprinkle with salt, pepper, and the dash of cayenne, and bake for 30 minutes.
5. Meanwhile, chop the onion and tomatoes into small pieces and drain the beans.
6. Toss the beans, tomatoes, and onion in a large bowl with the spices.
7. Once the chicken has cooked, chop or shred it into pieces and mix it with everything else.
8. This is fabulous as is, or serve in a warm corn tortilla.

Tasty Variations

➤ For a refreshing cold salad that keeps well in the fridge, tear up some romaine and toss with the inchilotta once it cools completely. Or, roll up the inchilotta mix in a lettuce leaf for healthy mini burritos.

➤ For a hot enchilada casserole, place a layer of corn tortillas in an oiled 9-x-7-inch baking dish. Cover with the enchilada mixture and then a layer of grated cheddar cheese. Top with another layer of tortillas and another sprinkling of cheese. Bake for 15 minutes at 350°F.

Cold Noodle Salad

Fresh and fantastic, this flavorful Asian-inspired dish is perfect for languid summer days, or any other time.

PREP: 15 minutes

COOKING: 15 minutes

TOTAL TIME: 15 minutes

YIELD: 6 cups

2 cups gluten-free spaghetti
3 carrots
2 green onions
1 cup green beans
¼ cup toasted sesame oil
2 tablespoons tamari
2 teaspoons agave nectar
1 teaspoon ground ginger
Dash cayenne
1 cup bean sprouts

1. This is a great way to use leftover pasta—you will need 2 cups of cooked, plain noodles. If you don't already have cooked noodles, they can cook while you prepare the rest of the dish. Use your favorite gluten-free spaghetti noodles, or try noodles made from quinoa. Use about 1½-inch-diameter's worth of dry noodles. Break them in half before cooking.
2. Thinly slice the carrots and green onions, and chop the green beans into 1-inch pieces. Set aside.
3. For the dressing, whisk together the sesame oil, tamari, agave, ginger, and cayenne. Or, you can put the ingredients in a jar and vigorously shake it up.
4. If you have just cooked the noodles, drain them and put them in the freezer for about 5 minutes to cool down. Once they are chilled, put them in a large bowl. If you are using leftover noodles, place them, cold, into a large bowl. Slice through the noodles several times so the strands are not very long.
5. Put the chopped vegetables and the bean sprouts in the bowl with the noodles and toss.
6. Pour on the dressing and mix well.

Veggie Sushi

These vegetarian rollups are easy to make and fun to eat. Filled with bright colors and gorgeous flavors, they quickly become addicting.

PREP: 10 minutes

COOKING: None

TOTAL TIME: 10 minutes

YIELD: 8 nori cones

2 carrots
½ cucumber
2 shallots
½ red bell pepper
1 cup alfalfa sprouts
2 nori sheets
1 avocado

1. Peel the carrots and the cucumber. Use the peeler to make ribbons of the carrots, or chop them into thin slivers. Slice the cucumber, shallots, and bell pepper into thin strips.
2. Cut the nori sheets into quarters, to make four small squares from each sheet.
3. Leaving a slight edge of nori along one side, smear some avocado on each square.
4. Arrange vegetables in the center of the nori, diagonally.
5. Roll the nori square diagonally to create a cone shape. Moisten the edge of the nori to seal it.
6. Top with a spray of sprouts.

HINT

Mix wasabi paste with tamari for a spicy dipping sauce.

Broccoli Lentil Pilaf

This hearty, autumnal meal is guaranteed to provide you with tons of energy and nutrition. Leftovers are especially good.

PREP: 5 minutes

COOKING: 1⅓ hours

TOTAL TIME: 1⅓ hours

YIELD: 6 cups

¾ cup dried lentils
½ cups brown rice
2 cups broccoli florets
¾ cup cheddar cheese, grated
½ teaspoon dried thyme
½ teaspoon dried basil
½ teaspoon sea salt
4 eggs
1 cup plain soy milk

1. *To cook the lentils:* Rinse the lentils and put into a pot with 1½ cups of water. Bring to a boil, then turn down the heat, cover, and simmer for 30 minutes. Do not add salt to the water, as it will toughen the lentils.
2. *To cook the brown rice:* Rinse the brown rice and put into a pot with 1 cup of water and 1 tablespoon of olive oil. Bring to a boil, then turn down the heat, cover, and simmer for 40 minutes.
3. Once the rice and lentils have cooked, preheat the oven to 350°F.
4. Chop the broccoli florets into small pieces. In a large bowl, mix the lentils, rice, broccoli, cheese, thyme, basil, and salt.
5. Oil an 8-inch square baking dish and fill with the lentil mixture.
6. In a small bowl, whisk the eggs and soy milk with a fork and pour this over the lentil mixture.
7. Top with a sprinkling of grated cheese and bake for 40 to 45 minutes.

Zucchini Pasta

This recipe will change your life and become an inevitable favorite. The leftovers are incredible, though there never seem to be any.

PREP: 15 minutes

COOKING: None

TOTAL TIME: 15 minutes

YIELD: 8 cups

4 medium-sized zucchini
3 tomatoes
⅓ cup Kalamata olives
⅓ cup fresh basil
1 clove garlic
2 tablespoons olive oil
1 teaspoon sea salt
½ teaspoon black pepper

1. To create the zucchini "pasta," use the fine attachment on a mandoline and slice the zucchini lengthwise to create long strands that mimic angel hair pasta. If you don't have a mandoline, you can use a vegetable peeler to make long ribbons out of the entire zucchini.
2. Chop the tomatoes, olives, and basil, and mince or press the garlic. Toss everything together in a large serving bowl. Drizzle with olive oil and season with salt and pepper. Toss again and taste.

WHAT'S A MANDOLINE?

A mandoline is a very sharp instrument with interchangeable blades that makes slicing and shredding vegetables super easy and quite beautiful. It can also cut your fingers, so be very, very careful. They range greatly in price, but all do pretty much the same thing. I have found the freestanding ones are easier to use and therefore safer. You can find them at most kitchen stores or online.

Quinoa Medley

Earthy and textural, quinoa is a fabulous source of protein. Traditional Latin American flavors infuse this filling and nutritious dish. It is delicious warm or cold.

PREP: 5 minutes

COOKING: 20 minutes

TOTAL TIME: 20 minutes

YIELD: 6 cups

1 cup quinoa
1 poblano chili
1½ cups vegetable broth
¾ teaspoon cinnamon
1 15-ounce can black beans (about 2 cups)
1 cob of corn (or about 1 cup frozen or canned corn)
1 tomato
1 red bell pepper
Dash hot sauce (optional)

1. Rinse the quinoa in a strainer and chop the poblano. Put the quinoa, poblano, broth, and cinnamon in a pot over high heat and bring to a boil.
2. Once it reaches a boil, cover the pot, turn down the heat, and let it simmer for 15 minutes.
3. Meanwhile, drain the black beans and put them in a large bowl.
4. Slice the corn off the cob—you can slice the kernels right off the cob directly into the bowl. Chop the tomato and bell pepper and add them to the bowl.
5. Once the quinoa has cooked, add it to the bowl as well.
6. Toss everything together and hit it with a little hot sauce if you like.

Polenta Pizza Pie

A new comfort food is born with this soft baked polenta, filled with gooey cheese, warm tomatoes, and any gluten-free pizza toppings you want.

PREP: 15 minutes

COOKING: 20 minutes

TOTAL TIME: 45 minutes

YIELD: 5 cups

1 18-ounce tube of precooked polenta
1–2 tablespoons water
1 cup canned crushed tomatoes
½ cup button or cremini mushrooms
½ cup spinach
1 cup fontinella or mozzarella cheese, grated

1. Preheat the oven to 350°F.
2. Break the polenta into big pieces and put them in a bowl. Warm the polenta in the microwave or the oven for just a few moments to soften it.
3. Add enough water to mash the polenta with a fork to a fairly smooth but thick consistency.
4. Stir the crushed tomatoes into the polenta. Slice the mushrooms, tear up the spinach, and stir into the polenta mixture with ½ cup of the grated cheese.
5. Spoon the mixture into a pie pan (or any baking dish), and top with the remaining cheese.
6. Bake for 20 minutes, until the cheese is bubbly and the pie is heated through.

Tasty Variation

Customize this as you would a regular pizza. Stir in sausage, black olives, anchovies . . . you're in charge.

Baked Swordfish

Classic Italian flavors meld with rich, mild swordfish. An easy, elegant meal.

PREP: 10 minutes

COOKING: 25 minutes

TOTAL TIME: 35 minutes

YIELD: Four ½-pound fillets

2 tomatoes
2 shallots
2 cloves garlic
3 tablespoons olive oil
2 teaspoons lemon juice
1 teaspoon dried oregano
1 teaspoon sea salt
½ teaspoon pepper
2 pounds swordfish steak

1. Preheat the oven to 400°F.
2. Chop the tomatoes and the shallots, and mix with the garlic, olive oil, lemon juice, oregano, salt, and pepper in a bowl.
3. Cut the fish into four equal pieces, and tear off four large squares of tinfoil. With the back of a spoon, coat the top and sides of each piece of fish with oil from the tomato-herb mixture, so that the fish will not stick to the foil. Put the fish, oiled side down, in the center of the foil.
4. Mound a generous amount of the tomato-herb mixture over the top of the fish.
5. Fold over the foil and close with a double fold to ensure that it is well sealed. Fold or twist the ends close to make a little package.
6. Place the foil-wrapped fish directly on the oven rack, and bake for 25 minutes.
7. Carefully unwrap the foil and transfer the delicious contents to a plate.

Ancient Millet Harvest

Warm and gentle, this subtle and satisfying dish is easy on the digestive system while providing lasting energy.

PREP: 5 minutes

COOKING: 30 minutes

TOTAL TIME: 35 minutes

YIELD: 6 cups

1 cup whole millet
2 cups chicken or vegetable broth
2 yellow squash (about 3 cups cut into chunks)
2 zucchini (about 2 cups cut into chunks)
1 clove garlic
2 tablespoons olive oil
½ teaspoon sea salt
½ teaspoon pepper

1. Put the millet and broth into a pot on the stove over high heat. Once it reaches a boil, cover the pot and turn down the heat to low. Simmer for 30 minutes.
2. Slice the squash and zucchini into ½-inch rounds, then cut each round into quarters.
3. When the millet has 10 minutes left to cook, put the squash and zucchini in a pot and steam for 5 minutes or until tender (see page 121).
4. Once the millet has cooked, put it in a large bowl and mix it with the garlic, olive oil, salt, and pepper.
5. Add the steamed zucchini and squash, and toss well.

Tasty Variation

Add a little romance to this dish with artichoke hearts. Stir them in at the end with the garlic. Mmmm.

Pizza

Now there's no need to pine away for pizza. In the time it takes to wait for delivery, you can toss one yourself.

PREP: 15 minutes

COOKING: 15 minutes

TOTAL TIME: 30 minutes

YIELD: 1 pizza

1 6-ounce can tomato paste
1 green pepper
1 small yellow onion
2 cups sliced mushrooms
½ cup sliced black olives
2 cups grated white cheddar cheese

1. First you must have some dough. See page 88 for the recipe.
2. Preheat the oven to 350°F.
3. Grease a cookie sheet and put the pizza crust on it.
4. Chop the green pepper and onion into small pieces or thin strips. Cover the crust with sauce and toppings.
5. Bake the pizza for 10 to 20 minutes, depending on thickness of the crust. Test by carefully lifting the edge of the pizza with a spatula to peek at the underside of the crust—it should be a light golden brown.

Tasty Variations

Pesto Pizza: Spread dough with 1 cup pesto. Cover with sliced tomatoes and mozzarella cheese.

BBQ Pizza: Spread dough with 1 cup barbeque sauce and cover with shredded chicken, red onion, and cilantro.

USING FROZEN PIZZA DOUGH

If you're using a frozen, unbaked crust, take it out of the freezer and allow it to thaw while you prepare the toppings. It *must* thaw completely for the yeast to "wake up" and make a fluffy crust. Put it on a greased cookie sheet, cover with toppings, and bake according to the preceding directions.

Poblanos Perfectos

Easy, delicious, and impressive—this is a great "show-off" meal for entertaining. Or, if you're dining alone, they're good enough to eat all week long.

PREP: 12 minutes

COOKING: 20 minutes

TOTAL TIME: 32 minutes

YIELD: 6 stuffed peppers

1 cob sweet corn (or ½ cup of canned corn)
1 15-ounce can black beans
1 4-ounce can mild green chilies
½ teaspoon sea salt
4 shakes hot sauce
3 poblano chilies
6 ounces soft Mexican cheese, such as ranchero or cotija

1. Preheat the oven to 350°F.
2. With a sharp knife, slice the raw kernels of corn off the cob and into a bowl.
3. Drain the black beans and add them to corn, along with the mild green chilies, sea salt, and the hot sauce, if desired. Mix everything together.
4. Cut the poblanos in half lengthwise, and remove the seeds and pith.
5. Spoon the bean and corn mixture into each of the six chili halves, and place them in a baking dish or pie pan.
6. Crumble the cheese on top of each stuffed pepper, lightly pressing it into the mixture.
7. Bake for 20 minutes.

Tasty Variation

Add 1 cup of cooked rice to the beans and corn. This will give you enough filling for four chilies.

Nightshade Sauté

This stovetop feast will warm you and fill you up.

PREP: 5 minutes

COOKING: 20 minutes

TOTAL TIME: 25 minutes

YIELD: 4 cups

1 pound new potatoes (very small red potatoes)
1 eggplant
½ yellow onion
1 clove garlic
2 tablespoons olive oil
1 15-ounce can crushed tomatoes
½ teaspoon sea salt
¼ teaspoon black pepper

1. Put the potatoes into a pot of water and boil for about 10 minutes. They are done when easily pierced with a knife.
2. Peel the eggplant and cut it into small cubes.
3. Chop the onion. Heat the oil in a pan and sauté the garlic and onions for about 5 minutes.
4. Roughly slice the boiled potatoes and add them to the pan with the eggplant. Sauté to lightly brown.
5. Stir in the crushed tomatoes, salt, and pepper, and allow it to gently simmer for about 5 minutes.

Tasty Variation

Top with a flavorful Italian cheese, such as fontina.

Shish Kebabs

These are so fun to make! So fun to eat! And you don't need a BBQ grill.

PREP: 15 minutes

COOKING: 10 minutes

TOTAL TIME: 25 minutes

YIELD: 8 shish kebabs

1 pound sirloin, rib eye steak, or chicken breast
Lemon Herb Marinade (page 174) or Teriyaki Marinade (page 175)
2 yellow onions
2 bell peppers
½ pound broccoli
10 button or cremini mushrooms
½ pint cherry tomatoes
Metal skewers

1. Cut the meat into chunks about 1½ inches square. Scissors make this easy.
2. Mix the marinade of your choice, add the meat, and place in the fridge for 10 minutes.
3. While the meat marinates, chop the onions into wedges, the bell peppers into large chunks, and the broccoli into florets. Leave the mushrooms and cherry tomatoes whole.
4. After the meat has soaked for 10 minutes, assemble the shish kebabs and drizzle them with the remaining marinade.
5. Lay the shish kebabs on a cookie sheet lined with foil. Put the oven rack in the topmost position, and set the oven to broil. Leave the oven door partly open while broiling.
6. Broil the shish kebabs for 6 minutes, then carefully flip them over and continue to broil for 4 minutes (with the oven door still open).

Quesadillas

Quesadillas are a great old standby. Easy to prepare with endless variation, you just can't go wrong with this Mexican favorite.

PREP: 2 minutes

COOKING: 4 minutes

TOTAL TIME: 6 minutes each

YIELD: 3 quesadillas

3 ounces white cheddar cheese
3 button mushrooms
1 shallot
6 corn tortillas

1. Grate the cheese or slice it thinly. Slice the mushrooms and chop the shallot.
2. Arrange some cheese on a corn tortilla, keeping it away from the edge, as the cheese will spread as it melts. Add a layer of onion and mushroom slices, then top with another tortilla.
3. Place it in a frying pan and warm over medium heat so the cheese will melt before the tortillas char. Flip to crisp the other side.
4. Slide it onto a plate and cut in half.
5. Repeat as many times as you like.

Tasty Variation

Be simple or get fancy—fill with spinach, tomato, meat, or diced vegetables—whatever your whim may be. Try other cheeses—Monterey Jack, ranchero, mozzarella, cheddar, on and on . . .

Tofu Cauli Curry

The warm, smoky flavors of curry dominate this delicious, healthy dish.

PREP: 5 minutes

COOKING: 20 minutes

TOTAL TIME: 25 minutes

YIELD: 6 cups

1 pound firm tofu
4 cups cauliflower
2 tablespoons olive oil
1 yellow onion
1 clove garlic
1 cup crushed tomatoes
2 cups chicken or vegetable broth
4 teaspoons curry powder

1. Cut the tofu into cubes and break the cauliflower into small pieces.
2. Heat the olive oil in a large saucepan. Chop the onion and sauté with the garlic.
3. Add the tofu and brown it on all sides for about 5 minutes.
4. Stir in the tomatoes, broth, curry powder, and cauliflower. Cook, simmering, for about 12 minutes until the liquid has reduced and the cauliflower is tender.

Tamales

For a fun party or family gathering, tamales are a hot idea. Have the dough ready, and let everyone make their own tamale.

PREP: 20 minutes

COOKING: 20 minutes

TOTAL TIME: 40 minutes

YIELD: 12 tamales

4 cups masa harina (traditional Mexican corn flour)
2 teaspoons sea salt
¼ cup olive oil
2½ cups water, or chicken or vegetable broth

Tamale filling:
1½ cups black beans
¼ cup mild green chilies
¼ cup diced tomatoes
1 teaspoon sea salt
½ teaspoon ground cumin
⅛ teaspoon cayenne
1 cup shredded chicken, prepared as on page 141
½ cup grated cheese

1. *To make the dough:* Mix the flour, salt, and oil in a large bowl.
2. Stir in the water or broth, ¼ cup at a time.
3. Once the dough is mixed, knead it for a few minutes. It will feel like Play-Doh.
4. *To make the filling:* Stir the black beans, chilies, tomatoes, and spices together. You may stir the cheese and chicken into this mixture as well, or keep separate for people to add as they wish.
5. *To make the tamales:* Tear off a square of tinfoil. Take a piece of dough that is about the size of an egg. Flatten it onto the tinfoil and roll out to ¼ inch. Use a bottle if you don't have a rolling pin.
6. Put about 2 heaping tablespoons of filling on one-half of the dough, leaving space at the edges. Fold over the tamale dough and press the edges together to seal it. (The first few might be ugly, but they will still taste good.)
7. Roll it up tightly in the tinfoil. Twist or fold the ends of the tinfoil to make an airtight tamale capsule.

8. Steam the wrapped tamales as you would steam vegetables, covered, for 20 minutes.

9. Keep wrapped until ready to eat.

HINT

These are a great item to freeze and nuke. Make them, steam them, and then freeze them. Remove the tinfoil before freezing unless you plan to reheat them in the oven.

Pasta Salad

A delicate delectable lemon dill delight, this Greek salad is fabulous warm or cold.

PREP: 10 minutes

COOKING: 20 minutes

TOTAL TIME: 30 minutes

YIELD: 8 cups

2 chicken breasts
2 cups gluten-free spiral pasta
2 tomatoes
½ English cucumber
2 shallots
1 green bell pepper
½ cup Kalamata or black olives
½ cup olive oil
¼ cup red wine vinegar
2 tablespoons lemon juice
1 clove garlic
½ teaspoon dill
½ teaspoon sea salt
½ teaspoon black pepper

1. Preheat the oven to 350°F.
2. Line a cookie sheet with tinfoil and lightly coat with oil. Place the chicken breasts on the sheet and bake for 20 to 25 minutes. You can tell the chicken is done by cutting into it—the juices should run clear.
3. Meanwhile, put water on to boil for the pasta. When it reaches a boil, add the pasta and cook until al dente, about 7 minutes.
4. Chop the tomatoes, cucumber (you can leave the skin on English cucumbers), shallots, green pepper, and olives; put everything in a large bowl.
5. Make the dressing by whisking together the olive oil, vinegar, lemon juice, garlic, dill, salt, and pepper.
6. Once the chicken has cooked, cut it into pieces. Add the chicken and the pasta to the bowl of vegetables and toss together.
7. Drizzle with the dressing and stir to coat everything. (You may have dressing left over.)

Tasty Variation

You can make a delicious vegetarian version by simply omitting the chicken.

SWEETS

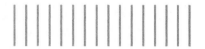

*Enjoy this tasty variety of treats and desserts,
many of which are dairy free as well as gluten free.
All of these sweets are simple to make
and delicious to eat.*

Chocolate Chip Cookie Bars

These are like good old chocolate chip cookies, but with the moist richness of a brownie. Yum.

PREP: 15 minutes

COOKING: 15 minutes

TOTAL TIME: 30 minutes

YIELD: 16 bars

1 cup sorghum flour
¼ cup millet flour
¾ teaspoon baking soda
¼ teaspoon salt
½ teaspoon xanthan gum
½ cup butter, softened
½ cup brown sugar
¼ cup granulated sugar
1 teaspoon vanilla
1 egg
1 cup chocolate chips

1. Preheat the oven to 375°F.
2. Mix the sorghum flour, millet flour, baking soda, salt, and xanthan gum, and set aside.
3. In a large bowl, whip together the softened butter, brown sugar, and granulated sugar.
4. Add the vanilla and the egg and beat well, until creamy and light.
5. Gradually stir in the flour mixture, about ½ cup at a time. Once mixed, stir in the chocolate chips.
6. Spoon the batter into an ungreased 8-inch square pan and bake for 15 minutes.
7. Allow to cool slightly, then cut into bars.

Fruit Crisp

Easier than pie! Fresh warm fruit nestles below a crumbly, caramel-ly crust. This crisp is so good you will be tempted to bake another one as soon as you finish the first!

PREP: 15 minutes

COOKING: 30 minutes

TOTAL TIME: 45 minutes

YIELD: 6 cups

5 cups fresh fruit, such as blueberries, apples, peaches, or plums
¼ cup granulated sugar
1 tablespoon cornstarch
1 cup chopped walnuts
¼ cup sorghum flour
¼ cup millet flour
½ cup brown sugar
1 teaspoon ground cinnamon
¼ teaspoon ground ginger
¼ teaspoon salt
6 tablespoons butter, softened

1. Preheat the oven to 400°F.
2. Cut the fruit into bite-size pieces and mix it with the granulated sugar and the cornstarch.
3. Put the fruit mixture into a baking dish. A glass bread pan is ideal; an 8-inch square or round casserole dish also works well.
4. Mix the walnuts, flour, brown sugar, and spices together in a bowl. Mix in the softened butter with a fork or with your fingers.
5. Arrange the mixture evenly over the top of the fruit. Bake for 30 minutes, until the top is browned and the fruit is bubbling.

HINT

Peaches and apples can be used with their skin on or off. Peel apples with a carrot peeler. To peel a peach, boil water in a large pot and, once the water is boiling, submerge the peach for one minute. Remove from the water and the skin will easily slide off.

Panna Cotta

This decadent dairy-free custard is subtle, creamy, and oh so rich.

PREP: 5 minutes

COOKING: 10 minutes

TOTAL TIME: 15 minutes, plus setting time

YIELD: 4 cups

3 tablespoons cold water
1 ¼-ounce packet unflavored gelatin
2 cups almond milk
2 cups coconut milk (do *not* use light or sweetened coconut milk)
¼ cup sugar
¼ teaspoon vanilla

1. Measure the water into a large bowl, sprinkle the gelatin evenly over it, and set this aside.
2. In a saucepan, mix the almond milk, coconut milk (shake the can of coconut milk before opening it), sugar, and vanilla. Bring to a simmer, stirring constantly.
3. Once it begins to simmer, remove from heat. Let it sit for about 5 minutes to slightly cool.
4. Pour ½ cup of the mixture into the bowl with the gelatin, and stir to dissolve the gelatin completely. Add the rest of the milk and stir it well.
5. Ladle into small cups or dishes. Put them in the fridge to set, about 1½ hours. This is divine with fresh fruit.

EZPBs

These rich, buttery peanut butter cookies are ridiculously simple to make. The batter keeps well in the fridge, to turn into warm cookies whenever the mood strikes.

PREP: 5 minutes

COOKING: 10 minutes

TOTAL TIME: 15 minutes

YIELD: 10 cookies

1 egg
½ cup sugar
⅓ cup butter
1 cup peanut butter
½ cup sorghum flour

1. Preheat the oven to 350ºF.
2. Beat the egg, sugar, and butter together. This is easy to do with a fork if the butter is slightly soft.
3. Add the peanut butter and mix well. Then stir in the flour.
4. Fashion into balls, place on an ungreased cookie sheet, and flatten with a fork.
5. Bake for 10 minutes.

Double Dark Chocolate Pudding

The name says it all—an indulgent and easy-to-make chilled pudding.

PREP: 3 minutes
COOKING: 10 minutes
TOTAL TIME: 13 minutes
YIELD: 3 cups

¾ cup sugar
⅓ cup cocoa
⅓ cup cornstarch
¼ teaspoon salt
3 cups chocolate rice milk

1. Put all the ingredients into a pot over medium heat.
2. Whisk together and continue to whisk while the pudding cooks. The pudding will soon thicken, darken, and begin to bubble.
3. Keep whisking while it bubbles for 30 seconds, then remove the pot from the stove and continue to stir for 30 seconds more.
4. Pour into serving cups and chill to set.
5. Enjoy as is, or top with whipped cream or raspberries.

Tasty Variation

Substitute almond milk for the chocolate rice milk.

Truffles

These treats alone make buying a food processor worthwhile. Yum! Try not to O.D. on them.

PREP: 8 minutes

COOKING: None

TOTAL TIME: 8 minutes

YIELD: 10 truffles

1 cup raw pecans
6 large Medjool dates
¼ cup coconut flakes
1 tablespoon cocoa powder or carob

1. Grind the pecans into small bits in a food processor with the S-blade.
2. Tear the dates in half, remove the pits, and put the dates in the food processor. Process with the pecans until they become incorporated.
3. Take some of this mixture and roll it in your hands to form a small ball. Repeat to use up all the mixture.
4. Roll some of the balls in the coconut flakes, some in the cocoa or carob, and leave some plain.
5. Chill briefly in the fridge.

Hippie Bars

Wondering what to make? Make these! Part cookie, part cake, these delicious snacks are packed with tons of nutritious treats.

PREP: 15 minutes

COOKING: 15 minutes

TOTAL TIME: 30 minutes

YIELD: 16 bars

¼ cup butter
1 cup sorghum flour
¼ cup millet flour
¾ teaspoon baking soda
½ teaspoon xanthan gum
¼ teaspoon salt
1 teaspoon ground cinnamon
½ teaspoon ground nutmeg
¼ cup applesauce
⅓ cup honey
1 egg
1 cup dried apricots or nectarines
1 cup unsweetened coconut flakes
½ cup chopped walnuts

1. Preheat the oven to 375°F.
2. Put the butter into a small dish and put it in the oven to melt, or use a microwave.
3. In a large bowl, mix the sorghum flour, millet flour, baking soda, xanthan gum, salt, cinnamon, and nutmeg together.
4. Stir the applesauce, butter, and honey into the flour mix once the butter has cooled off a bit—don't add it if it's still hot. Add the egg and mix well.
5. Chop the dried fruit into small bits, and stir into the batter with the coconut and walnuts.
6. Spoon the batter into an 8-inch square pan and bake for 15 minutes. These make pretty amazing muffins, too.

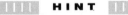

HINT

When measuring honey, coat the measuring cup or spoon with a touch of vegetable oil before using it for the honey. The honey will slide right out and leave no sticky mess at all.

Macaroons

These gooey coconut cookies are sure to satisfy any sweet tooth.

PREP: 5 minutes

COOKING: 15 minutes

TOTAL TIME: 20 minutes

YIELD: 15 macaroons

2½ cups shredded coconut
⅓ cup sugar
⅛ teaspoon salt
3 tablespoons gluten-free flour
2 egg whites
½ teaspoon vanilla

1. Preheat the oven to 350°F.
2. Mix the coconut, sugar, salt, and flour together.
3. In a separate bowl, froth up the egg whites with a fork. Add the vanilla to the egg whites, then stir into the coconut mixture.
4. Drop spoonfuls onto a cookie sheet lined with parchment paper.
5. Bake for 15 minutes, until golden brown.

HINT

Most gluten-free flours are suitable for this recipe: sorghum, millet, tapioca, rice, premixed flours—use your favorite, or whatever you have around. Avoid corn, soy, garbanzo, and quinoa, however, as their flavors are too powerful.

Energy Nuggets

Crunchy, creamy, nutty, yummy, these delectable trail mix treats are packed with great flavors and loads of nutrition.

PREP: 10 minutes	1 cup almond butter
COOKING: None	1 cup nutty rice cereal
TOTAL TIME: 10 minutes, plus chilling	⅔ cup coconut flakes
YIELD: 20 nuggets	⅔ cup dried apricots, nectarines, or raisins
	½ cup chocolate chips
	¼ cup sesame seeds

1. Stir the almond butter and rice cereal together in a large bowl.
2. Add the coconut flakes. Chop the dried apricots, nectarines, or raisins and add to the mix, along with the chocolate chips.
3. Place the sesame seeds in a separate bowl and set aside.
4. Form the mixture into little nugget shapes and roll in the sesame seeds to coat.
5. Place on a plate and put into the freezer to chill for a while. You can store these in the freezer or the fridge, whichever you prefer.

HINT

You can often find nutty rice cereal in the bulk section of a health food store.

Sugar Meringues

These are not instant-gratification cookies—they "cook" overnight. But they are so fun and yummy, they are worth the wait.

PREP: 10 minutes

COOKING: Overnight

TOTAL TIME: 10 minutes + overnight

YIELD: 16 meringues

2 egg whites
⅔ cup sugar

1. Preheat the oven to 250°F.
2. Line a cookie sheet with waxed paper or parchment paper.
3. Beat the egg whites until soft peaks form.
4. Gradually add the sugar while beating the egg whites. Keep beating until the mixture holds stiff peaks.
5. Drop spoonfuls of meringue onto the lined cookie sheet.
6. Put the meringues in the oven and *turn the oven off.* Leave them in there overnight. No sneak previews allowed (i.e., don't open the oven door).
7. In the morning, carefully peel the meringues off the waxed paper and store in an airtight container.

Tasty Variations

After the sugar is mixed into the egg whites, you can add chocolate chips, mint chocolate chips, crushed up candy canes, or anything else you can think of and want to try. Or mix in drops of food coloring of all different colors and shades. Get ready for a sugar trip.

HINT

These go over really well at parties, and they are really easy to mass-produce—just double the ingredients.

Halvah

This simple confection is a blend of honey, cocoa, and tahini, a nut butter made from sesame seeds. Tahini has a very distinct acrid flavor that gives this sweet stuff some dimension. It's addicting.

PREP: 7 minutes

COOKING: None

TOTAL TIME: 7 minutes

YIELD: 20 pieces

1 cup tahini
¼ cup unsweetened cocoa or carob
   powder
½ to ¾ cup honey

1. In a small bowl, stir the cocoa into the tahini.
2. Vigorously stir in ½ cup of honey. Slowly add more honey until you reach your desired level of sweetness.
3. Roll into balls and store in the fridge.

Date Tart

A rich, nutty crust forms the perfect foundation for soft vibrant fruit. Your tongue will flip.

PREP: 10 minutes

COOKING: 10 minutes

TOTAL TIME: 20 minutes

YIELD: 1 large pie or tart crust or
    4 individual tarts or 8 tiny tartlets

2 cups raw pecans
5 large Medjool dates
1 tablespoon orange juice
4 apricots
4 kiwi
½ cup fresh raspberries

1. Preheat the oven to 275°F.
2. Grind the pecans in a food processor with the S-blade until fairly fine.
3. Tear the dates in half, remove the pits, and put the dates in the food processor. Process to integrate them into the pecan flour.
4. Add the orange juice and process. It will form a ball of dough.
5. Take this mixture and press into a pie pan or tart pan. Or you can make mini tarts by modeling them free-form. Make any shape you like and pinch the edges up to form the sides. If free-forming, make them right onto a cookie sheet.
6. Stab the bottom of the pie crust or the little tart shells with a fork once or twice.
7. Bake for 10 minutes to firm the outside of the crust while keeping the insides moist.
8. After it has cooked, arrange a rainbow of apricot and kiwi slices in the crust and dapple with raspberries.

MARINADES
AND DRESSINGS

||||||||||||||||

*Keep your taste buds entertained
with these scrumptious salad dressings and
easy marinades. Commercial marinades
and dressings can be a source of hidden gluten,
so shake up your own.*

Lemon Herb Marinade

Marinades are a simple way to infuse flavor into meat before cooking. These flavors are fresh and bright, perfect for chicken or fish.

PREP: 5 minutes

YIELD: ½ cup

½ cup lemon juice
½ yellow onion, sliced in thin rings
1 teaspoon thyme or basil
1 clove garlic
½ teaspoon sea salt
½ teaspoon black pepper

1. Mix all the ingredients together in a bowl or shallow pan.
2. Add the meat and let it marinate in the fridge for at least 10 minutes or up to 2 hours.

HINT

This marinade is great with the Baked Chicken (page 137), Grilled Fish (page 139), and Shish Kebabs (page 153).

Teriyaki Marinade

Marinades are a simple way to infuse flavor into meat before cooking. A rich combination of earthy flavors makes this marinade delicious with steak, chicken, or fish.

PREP: 5 minutes

YIELD: ½ cup

½ cup tamari
1 tablespoon honey
1 tablespoon sesame oil
1 clove garlic
½ teaspoon black pepper
2 tablespoons fresh grated ginger
   (optional)

1. Mix all the ingredients together in a bowl or shallow pan.
2. Add the meat and let it marinate in the fridge for at least 10 minutes or up to 2 hours.

HINT

Try this tasty marinade with the Baked Chicken (page 137), Grilled Fish (page 139), Shish Kebabs (page 153), and One Great Steak (page 140).

Basic Balsamic Vinaigrette

Dynamic sparks of mustard and black pepper combine with delicious balsamic vinegar and mellow, rich olive oil to create this everyday favorite.

PREP: 5 minutes

YIELD: ¾ cup

½ cup olive oil
¼ cup balsamic vinegar
1 teaspoon mustard powder
½ teaspoon black pepper
Dash sea salt

1. The simplest way to make a great dressing is to use a jar with a screw-on lid to mix it in. Small mason jars, used for canning, are great; or wash and reuse something like an applesauce jar. Put all the dressing ingredients into the jar, screw on the lid, and shake it vigorously. Then you can store leftover dressing in the jar in the fridge.
2. Alternately, put all the ingredients in a bowl, and using a whisk, whip them together until creamy and smooth.

Sweet Rice Vinaigrette

Delicate spices play the leading role in this lovely sweet dressing.

PREP: 5 minutes

YIELD: ¾ cup

½ cup vegetable oil
¼ cup rice vinegar
2 teaspoons agave nectar
½ teaspoon coriander
1 teaspoon ginger
½ teaspoon salt

1. The simplest way to make a great dressing is to use a jar with a screw-on lid to mix it in. Small mason jars, used for canning, are great; or wash and reuse something like an applesauce jar. Put all the dressing ingredients into the jar, screw on the lid, and shake it vigorously. Then you can store leftover dressing in the jar in the fridge.
2. Alternately, put all the ingredients in a bowl, and using a whisk, whip them together until creamy and smooth.

Cumin Dressing

Bring a bit of sunshine to every bite with this light and bright dressing.

PREP: 5 minutes

YIELD: ¾ cup

½ cup olive oil
¼ cup + 2 tablespoons lemon juice
1 teaspoon ground cumin
¼ teaspoon sea salt
¼ teaspoon black pepper
Dash cayenne

1. The simplest way to make a great dressing is to use a jar with a screw-on lid to mix it in. Small mason jars, used for canning, are great; or wash and reuse something like an applesauce jar. Put all the dressing ingredients into the jar, screw on the lid, and shake it vigorously. Then you can store leftover dressing in the jar in the fridge.
2. Alternately, put all the ingredients in a bowl, and using a whisk, whip them together until creamy and smooth.

Honey Dijon Vinaigrette

This classic, creamy honey mustard combo is good enough to spread on toast.

PREP: 5 minutes

YIELD: ¾ cup

½ cup olive oil
¼ cup red wine vinegar or balsamic
    vinegar
2 tablespoons Dijon mustard
1 tablespoon honey
¼ teaspoon sea salt

1. The simplest way to make a great dressing is to use a jar with a screw-on lid to mix it in. Small mason jars, used for canning, are great; or wash and reuse something like an applesauce jar. Put all the dressing ingredients into the jar, screw on the lid, and shake it vigorously. Then you can store leftover dressing in the jar in the fridge.
2. Alternately, put all the ingredients in a bowl, and using a whisk, whip them together until creamy and smooth.

Tahini Dressing

So rich and nutty, this dressing can turn a salad into a meal.

PREP: 5 minutes

YIELD: ¾ cup

½ cup tahini
⅓ cup water
Juice of 1 lemon
1 clove garlic
½ teaspoon dill
½ teaspoon sea salt

1. Put all the ingredients together in a bowl.
2. Mix well with a fork.

Sesame Dressing

A smoky and smooth blend of deep sesame, sweet agave, citrus, and spice.

PREP: 5 minutes

YIELD: ¾ cup

½ cup toasted sesame oil
2 tablespoons tamari
2 tablespoons rice vinegar
2 tablespoons lemon, lime, or orange juice
1½ teaspoons agave nectar
½ teaspoon ginger
1 clove garlic

1. The simplest way to make a great dressing is to use a jar with a screw-on lid to mix it in. Small mason jars, used for canning, are great; or wash and reuse something like an applesauce jar. Put all the dressing ingredients into the jar, screw on the lid, and shake it vigorously. Then you can store leftover dressing in the jar you made it in, in the fridge.
2. Alternately, put all the ingredients in a bowl, and using a whisk, whip them together until creamy and smooth.

Citrus Dressing

This delicious sweet and spicy dressing is perfect for summer, or for when you just want it to be summer.

PREP: 5 minutes

YIELD: ¾ cup

½ cup vegetable oil
2 tablespoons red wine vinegar
1 tablespoon lemon juice
⅓ cup orange juice
1 teaspoon agave nectar
1 clove garlic
½ teaspoon cumin
½ teaspoon coriander
½ teaspoon sea salt
½ teaspoon pepper
Dash cayenne

1. The simplest way to make a great dressing is to use a jar with a screw-on lid to mix it in. Small mason jars, used for canning, are great; or wash and reuse something like an applesauce jar. Put all the dressing ingredients into the jar, screw on the lid, and shake it vigorously. Then you can store leftover dressing in the jar in the fridge.
2. Alternately, put all the ingredients in a bowl, and using a whisk, whip them together until creamy and smooth.

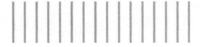

Resources

When you are dealing with gluten intolerance, knowledge is essential to stay safe, healthy, and sane. The issues you will confront are diverse and often complex, and the more you know, the better. It's important to take the time to learn as much as possible about gluten intolerance, espccially since so few doctors have an extensive understanding of the condition. Your health and well-being depend on your own initiative. The following resources are those I have found to be the most informative, the most well organized, and the most valuable. Explore them all and they will help facilitate the discovery of information, support, and gluten-free products.

National Celiac Associations

Gluten Intolerance Group
15110 10th Avenue SW, Suite A
Seattle, WA 98166
(206) 246-6652
Fax: (206) 246-6531
www.gluten.net
   A thorough and informative source.

Celiac Sprue Association
P.O. Box 31700
Omaha, NE 68131
(402) 558-0600
(877) 272-4272
www.csaceliacs.org

Canadian Celiac Association
5170 Dixie Road, Suite 204
Mississauga, Ontario L4W 1E3
Canada
(905) 507-6208
(800) 363-7296
Fax: (905) 507-4673
www.celiac.ca

Information and Support

Planet Celiac
www.planetceliac.com
   Very informative site, extensive and user-friendly. A good site to pass on to family and friends.

Gluten-free Diet Support Center
www.celiac.com
> The best way to find information on this site is to click the "Site Index" and choose links from there.

R.O.C.K. Raising Our Celiac Kids
www.celiackids.com
> Support and information for parents of celiac children.

Whole Foods Market
www.wholefoods.com
> A wealth of information on health, food, and nutrition. Try these links:
> Health Info > Health and Wellness Topics > Living Gluten-Free
> Health Info > Nutrition Reference Library

Online Health Forums

Maelstrom Listserv
http://maelstrom.stjohns.edu
> Choose "Online List Archives," then scroll down to find "celiac." From there you can access the Celiac/Gluten-Free archives and join the list.

> This was the single most helpful resource to me, especially during the first six months after my diagnosis. Their setup is extremely convenient: Once you register, you receive e-mail automatically from anyone who posts to the Listserv. These range from common and uncommon questions, to product alerts, to a general sharing of information and support. This is a fabulous passive way to learn an extraordinary amount of information, much of which you probably don't even know you need to know. Asking a question of the list involves simply sending one e-mail. You must register to receive e-mail, and to post questions. You may access the archives without becoming a member. I highly recommend this site.

Delphi Forums
www.delphiforums.com
> Type "celiac" or "gluten" in the search box. This will take you to the Celiac Forum, which has over 10,000 members.

> This resource provides gluten-free product lists, contacts for local support groups, articles, discussion forums, and their archives. You do not need to be a member to access this information, only to post.

BrainTalk Communities
www.braintalk.org
> Type "gluten" in the search box to find the Gluten Sensitivity/Celiac forum.

> This site is a bit difficult to navigate but can be helpful, as it focuses primarily on neurological issues. You do not need to be a member to access this information, only to post.

Online Retail Outlets for Gluten-Free Products

Gluten Solutions
8750 Concourse Court
San Diego, CA 92123
(888) 845-8836
www.glutensolutions.com

Gluten-Free Pantry
P.O. Box 840
Glastonbury, CT 06033
(860) 633-3826
(860) 633-6853 Fax
www.glutenfree.com

Gluten-Free Food Vendor Directory
www.gfmall.com
> Lists vendors and manufacturers of gluten-free products with links to their Web sites.

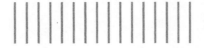

For Further Reading

Going Against the Grain: How Reducing and Avoiding Grains Can Revitalize Your Health
Melissa Diane Smith
McGraw-Hill Books
An exploration into the adverse effects that grains have upon the human body and mind, along with fascinating sociological insights.

Dangerous Grains: Why Gluten Cereal Grains May Be Hazardous to Your Health
James Braley, M.D., and Ron Hoggan, M.A.
Avery Penguin Putnam Books
Outlines the numerous physiological disorders and chronic ailments that are evidentially caused by gluten-based foods, and that can be reversed through changing what we eat.

Wheat-Free, Worry-Free: The Art of Happy, Healthy Gluten-Free Living
Danna Korn
Hay House Publishing
An easy-to-read guide for all matters gluten free. Informative and accessible.

Living Without
P.O. Box 2126
Northbrook, IL 60065
(847) 480-8810
www.livingwithout.com
A magazine focusing on food allergies; the Web site includes archived articles.

Gluten-Free Living
19A Broadway
Hawthorne, NY 10532
(914) 741-5420
www.glutenfreeliving.com
A quarterly magazine; addresses issues that confront those with gluten intolerance.

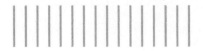

Acknowledgments

Ten thousand thanks
to all who have been involved.

My deepest gratitude to
Malia, Martha, Sue,
and Karin,
without whom this could not have
been accomplished.

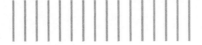

Index

almond butter, in Energy Nuggets, 168
Almond Cakes, 80
Almond Flour (Almond Milk variation), 75
Almond Milk, 75
    Double Dark Chocolate Pudding
        (variation), 164
    Panna Cotta, 162
    Polenta Breakfast Pudding, 52
Ancient Millet Harvest, 149
apples, in Fruit Crisp, 161
apples, in Power Punch, 66
apricots, dried
    Energy Nuggets, 168
    Hippie Bars, 166
apricots, fresh
    Date Tart, 171
    Green Tea Tonic, 70
    Mock Mimosas, 62
arrowroot, 25
artichoke hearts, in Ancient Millet Harvest
    (variation), 149
Artichokes, Steamed, 125
avocados
    Holy Guacamole, 132
    Salad Tepoz, 112
    Sexy Salad, 116
    Veggie Sushi, 143

Balsamic Sauté, 122
Balsamic Vinaigrette, Basic, 176
bananas
    Blue Banana Smoothie, 64
    Buckwheat Banana Bread, 79
    Coconut Bliss, 67
    Desert Dessert, 65
    Peanultimate Smoothie, 68
    Punch It Up, 60
    Super Deluxe Smoothie, 69
    Sweet Shake, 59
basil, in Power Pesto, 133
BBQ Pizza (variation), 150
beans and legumes
    black
        Huevos Rancheros, 49
        Inchilotta, 141
        Poblanos Perfectos, 151
        Quinoa Medley, 146
        Tamales, 156–157
    garbanzo, in Hummus, 131
    green, in Cold Noodle Salad, 142
    Lentils, 129
        Broccoli Lentil Pilaf, 144
        Lentil Soup, 108
    sprouts, in Cold Noodle Salad, 142
beef
    Hearty Beef Stew, 100

One Great Steak, 140
Shish Kebabs, 153
beets, in Roasted Roots, 123
Blue Banana Smoothie, 64
blueberries
    Blue Banana Smoothie, 64
    Fruit Crisp, 161
    Hot Cakes (variation), 48
breads
    Almond Cakes, 80
    baking tips, 78
    Buckwheat Banana Bread, 79
    Cinnamon Rolls, 50–51
    Cornbread, 83
    Hot Cakes, 48
    Hot Crossbread, 87
    Lace Crepes, 82
    Pizza Dough, 88–89
    Puff Rolls, 84–85
    Pumpkin Bread, 81
    Rosemary Focaccia, 90–91
    Sopas, 86
    Wheatish Bread, 92
Broccoli Lentil Pilaf, 144
Broccoli Soup, Creamy, 97
Brown Rice, 128
    Broccoli Lentil Pilaf, 144
    brown rice syrup, 24
buckwheat
    Buckwheat Banana Bread, 79
    flour, 25
    kasha, 24
buttermilk, in Smooth Smoothie, 73

carrots, in Roasted Roots, 123
Carrot Soup, 98
Cauli Curry, Tofu, 155
Cauliflower Soup, Creamy, 103
celiac disease, 11, 12–14
cheese
    Broccoli Lentil Pilaf, 144
    Huevos Rancheros, 49
    Inchilotta (variation), 141
    Nightshade Sauté (variation), 152
    Pizza, 150
    Poblanos Perfectos, 151
    Polenta Pizza Pie, 147
    Quesadillas, 154
    Strawberry Spinach Salad, 115

Tamales, 156–157
chicken
    Baked Chicken, 137
    BBQ Pizza (variation), 150
    Chicken Vegetable Soup, 95
    Inchilotta, 141
    Just Plain Chicken, 138
    Pasta Salad, 158
    Shish Kebabs, 153
    Tamales, 156–157
chilies, in Poblanos Perfectos, 151
chocolate
    Chocolate Chip Cookie Bars, 160
    Double Dark Chocolate Pudding, 164
    Energy Nuggets, 168
    Halvah, 170
    Heavenly Smoothie, 71
    Sugar Meringues (variation), 169
Cinnamon Rolls, 50–51
Citrus Dressing, 182
coconut
    Carrot Soup, 98
    Coconut Bliss, 67
    Energy Nuggets, 168
    Hippie Bars, 166
    Macaroons, 167
    Truffles, 165
    young, to open, 99
coconut milk, in Panna Cotta, 162
cookies
    Chocolate Chip Cookie Bars, 160
    EZPBs, 163
    Hippie Bars, 166
    Macaroons, 167
    Sugar Meringues, 169
cooking. See food and cooking
corn, in Poblanos Perfectos, 151
corn, in Quinoa Medley, 146
corn flour
    about, 25
    Sopas, 86
    Tamales, 156–157
    Wheatish Bread, 92
cornmeal and polenta
    about, 24, 25
    Cornbread, 83
    Polenta Breakfast Pudding, 52
    Polenta Pizza Pie, 147
cornstarch, 25

Crepes, Lace, 82
Crossbread, Hot, 87
Cukes, Sweet, 119
Cumin Dressing, 178
Curry, Tofu Cauli, 155

dairy intolerance, 14–15, 16
dates
    Date Tart, 171
    Desert Dessert, 65
    Nut Nog (Almond Milk variation), 75
    Truffles, 165
Desert Dessert, 65
desserts
    Chocolate Chip Cookie Bars, 160
    Date Tart, 171
    Double Dark Chocolate Pudding, 164
    Energy Nuggets, 168
    EZPBs, 163
    Fruit Crisp, 161
    Halvah, 170
    Hippie Bars, 166
    Panna Cotta, 162
    Sugar Meringues, 169
    sweetener substitutions, 38–39
    Truffles, 165
Dijon Honey Vinaigrette, 179
Double Dark Chocolate Pudding, 164
Dream Smoothie, Creamy, 61
dressings, salad. See salad dressings
drinks. See smoothies

eggplant, in Nightshade Sauté, 152
eggs
    Easiest Eggs, 53
    Huevos Rancheros, 49
    Italian Greens, 113
    Perfect Hard-Boiled Egg, 54
Energy Nuggets, 168
Exotic Steak Salad, 118

fats, substitutions for, 39
fish
    Baked Swordfish, 148
    Grilled Fish, 139
    Seafood Gumbo, 104–105
flaxseed meal, as fat substitute, 39
flaxseed meal, as supplement for
    smoothies, 56

flaxseed oil
    Heavenly Smoothie, 71
    Super Deluxe Smoothie, 69
    as supplement for smoothies, 56
flours. See also specific flours
    almond (Almond Milk variation), 75
    gluten-free, 25–26
    mixes, 78
Focaccia, Rosemary, 90–91
food and cooking
    enjoyment of cooking, 34–35
    equipment, 36–37
    farmers' markets, 41–42
    food storage, 39–40
    frozen foods
        convenience dinners, 136
        to freeze fruit, 57
        to thaw, 40
    glossary, 24–26
    herb gardens, 42
    measurements, 38
    spices, 37
    sprouts, 43–44
    substitutions, 38–39
Fruit Crisp, 161
fruits. See specific fruits

garbanzo beans, in Hummus, 131
Gazpacho, 109
gluten
    cross-contamination, 20–21
    gluten-free foods and foods containing,
        22–26
    hidden, 19–20
    reasons to avoid, 16–17
gluten-free lifestyle
    restaurants, 28–29
    social gatherings, 28, 30–32
    spiritual and emotional issues, 32–33
gluten intolerance
    celiac disease and related conditions,
        11–14
    dairy intolerance, 14–15
    healing process, 15
    sources of information and products,
        183–184
    symptoms and consequences, 9–10
    triggers, 8
grapefruit, in Punch It Up, 60

grapefruit, in Sunshine Salad, 114
green beans, in Cold Noodle Salad, 142
Greens, Italian, 113
greens, to store, 113
Green Tea Tonic, 70
Guacamole, Holy, 132

Halvah, 170
Hard-Boiled Egg, Perfect, 54
Heavenly Smoothie, 71
Hippie Bars, 166
Holy Guacamole, 132
honey, to measure, 78
Honey Dijon Vinaigrette, 179
Hot Cakes, 48
Huevos Rancheros, 49
Hummus, 131

Inchilotta, 141
Italian Greens, 113

jicama, in Summertime Salad, 117
Just Plain Chicken, 138

Kebabs, 153
kiwis, in Date Tart, 171

Lace Crepes, 82
Leek Potato Soup, 96
Lemon Herb Marinade, 174
Lentils, 129
    Broccoli Lentil Pilaf, 144
    Lentil Soup, 108

Macaroons, 167
mangoes
    Coconut Bliss, 67
    to peel, 116
    Sexy Salad, 116
Marinade, Lemon Herb, 174
Marinade, Teriyaki, 175
meats
    cuts for stews, 101
    Exotic Steak Salad, 118
    free-range, health benefits of, 33
    Hearty Beef Stew, 100
    One Great Steak, 140
    seasoned, gluten in, 24
    Shish Kebabs, 153

Meringues, Sugar, 169
milks
    Almond Milk, 75
        Double Dark Chocolate Pudding
            (variation), 164
        Panna Cotta, 162
        Polenta Breakfast Pudding, 52
    buttermilk, in Smooth Smoothie, 73
    coconut, in Panna Cotta, 162
    raw, for dairy intolerance, 14–15
    rice, in Double Dark Chocolate Pudding,
        164
    soy
        Blue Banana Smoothie, 64
        Creamy Broccoli Soup, 97
        Creamy Dream Smoothie, 61
        Desert Dessert, 65
        Heavenly Smoothie, 71
        Peanultimate Smoothie, 68
        Pumpkin Spice Smoothie, 74
        Sweet Shake, 59
    substitutions, 39
Millet, 127
millet flour
    about, 25
    Buckwheat Banana Bread, 79
    Chocolate Chip Cookie Bars, 160
    Fruit Crisp, 161
    Hippie Bars, 166
    Hot Cakes, 48
    Pumpkin Bread, 81
Millet Harvest, Ancient, 149
Mimosas, Mock, 62
mushrooms, for Grilled Portobellos, 120
Mushroom Tomato Soup, 106

nectarines, dried, in Energy Nuggets, 168
nectarines, dried, in Hippie Bars, 166
Nightshade Sauté, 152
Noodle Salad, Cold, 142
Nut Nog (Almond Milk variation), 75
nuts. See specific nuts

oats, cross-contamination in, 24
okra, in Seafood Gumbo, 104–105
One Great Steak, 140
oranges
    Mock Mimosas, 62
    Papaya Pond Sludge, 72

Punch It Up, 60
Sunshine Salad, 114
Super Deluxe Smoothie, 69

Panna Cotta, 162
papayas
    Exotic Steak Salad, 118
    Papaya Pond Sludge, 72
    Tropical Twist Smoothie, 58
parsnips, in Roasted Roots, 123
pasta, in Cold Noodle Salad, 142
Pasta, Zucchini, 145
Pasta Salad, 158
peaches
    Creamy Dream Smoothie, 61
    Fruit Crisp, 161
    Papaya Pond Sludge, 72
    to peel, 161
Peanultimate Smoothie, 68
peanut butter, in EZPBs, 163
pears, in Salad Tepoz, 112
pecans, in Date Tart, 171
pecans, in Truffles, 165
Pesto, Power, 133
Pesto Pizza (variation), 150
Pilaf, Broccoli Lentil, 144
pineapple
    Power Punch, 66
    Sunshine Salad, 114
    Tropical Twist Smoothie, 58
Pizza, 150
    Pizza Dough, 88–89
    Polenta Pizza Pie, 147
plums, in Fruit Crisp, 161
Poblanos Perfectos, 151
polenta
    about, 24
    Polenta Breakfast Pudding, 52
    Polenta Pizza Pie, 147
Portobellos, Grilled, 120
potatoes
    Nightshade Sauté, 152
    Potato Leek Soup, 96
    Steak Fries, 124
poultry. See chicken
Power Pesto, 133
Power Punch, 66
protein powder, as supplement for
    smoothies, 56

puddings
    Double Dark Chocolate Pudding, 164
    Panna Cotta, 162
    Polenta Breakfast Pudding, 52
Puff Rolls, 84–85
Pumpkin Bread, 81
Pumpkin Spice Smoothie, 74
Punch It Up, 60
Purely Vegetable Soup, 102

Quesadillas, 154
Quinoa, 126
Quinoa Medley, 146

raisins, in Energy Nuggets, 168
raspberries
    Date Tart, 171
    Heavenly Smoothie, 71
    Papaya Pond Sludge, 72
    Sweet Shake, 59
raw foods, benefits of, 17, 62
raw meat, gluten in, 24
rice
    Broccoli Lentil Pilaf, 144
    Brown Rice, 128
    glutinous, 24
    Poblanos Perfectos (variation), 151
    rice syrup, 24
    Wild Rice, 130
rice flour, 25
rice milk, in Double Dark Chocolate
        Pudding, 164
Rice Vinaigrette, Sweet, 177
Roots, Roasted, 123
Rosemary Focaccia, 90–91

salad dressings
    Basic Balsamic Vinaigrette, 176
    Citrus Dressing, 182
    Cumin Dressing, 178
    Honey Dijon Vinaigrette, 179
    Sesame Dressing, 181
    Sweet Rice Vinaigrette, 177
    Tahini Dressing, 180
    vinegars, 24
salads
    Cold Noodle Salad, 142
    Exotic Steak Salad, 118
    Inchilotta (variation), 141

Italian Greens, 113
Pasta Salad, 158
Salad Tepoz, 112
Sexy Salad, 116
Strawberry Spinach Salad, 115
Summertime Salad, 117
Sunshine Salad, 114
seafood, imitation, 24
Seafood Gumbo, 104–105
seaweed, in Miso Soup, 107
Sesame Dressing, 181
Sexy Salad, 116
shakes. *See* smoothies
Shish Kebabs, 153
shrimp, in Seafood Gumbo, 104–105
side dishes
    Balsamic Sauté, 122
    Brown Rice, 128
    Cooked Artichokes, 125
    Grilled Portobellos, 120
    Holy Guacamole, 132
    Hummus, 131
    Lentils, 129
    Millet, 127
    Power Pesto, 133
    Quinoa, 126
    Roasted Roots, 123
    Steak Fries, 124
    Steamed Veggies, 121
    Sweet Cukes, 119
    Wild Rice, 130
smoothies
    additions and supplements, 56
    Blue Banana Smoothie, 64
    Coconut Bliss, 67
    Creamy Dream Smoothie, 61
    Desert Dessert, 65
    Green Tea Tonic, 70
    Heavenly Smoothie, 71
    Mock Mimosas, 62
    Papaya Pond Sludge, 72
    Peanultimate Smoothie, 68
    Power Punch, 66
    Pumpkin Spice Smoothie, 74
    Punch It Up, 60
    Smooth Smoothie, 73
    Standard Smoothie, 57
    Super Deluxe Smoothie, 69
    Sweet Shake, 59

    tips for, 73
    Tropical Twist Smoothie, 58
    V-8000, 63
Sopas, 86
sorghum flour
    about, 26
    Chocolate Chip Cookie Bars, 160
    Cinnamon Rolls, 50–51
    EZPBs, 163
    Fruit Crisp, 161
    Hippie Bars, 166
    Hot Cakes, 48
    Hot Crossbread, 87
    Pizza Dough, 88–89
    Puff Rolls, 84–85
    Pumpkin Bread, 81
    Rosemary Focaccia, 90–91
    Wheatish Bread, 92
soups and stews
    Carrot Soup, 98
    Chicken Vegetable Soup, 95
    Creamy Broccoli Soup, 97
    Creamy Cauliflower Soup, 103
    Gazpacho, 109
    Hearty Beef Stew, 100
    Lentil Soup, 108
    Miso Soup, 107
    Mushroom Tomato Soup, 106
    Potato Leek Soup, 96
    Purely Vegetable Soup, 102
    Seafood Gumbo, 104–105
    to store, 95
soy flour
    about, 26
    Cornbread, 83
    Hot Crossbread, 87
soy milk
    Blue Banana Smoothie, 64
    Creamy Broccoli Soup, 97
    Creamy Dream Smoothie, 61
    Desert Dessert, 65
    Heavenly Smoothie, 71
    Peanultimate Smoothie, 68
    Pumpkin Spice Smoothie, 74
    Sweet Shake, 59
spices, essential, 37
spices, wheat flour in, 25
spinach
    Power Pesto, 133

Power Punch, 66
Strawberry Spinach Salad, 115
spirulina, as supplement for smoothies, 56
spirulina, in Super Deluxe Smoothie, 69
sprouts
Cold Noodle Salad, 142
to grow, 43–44
Salad Tepoz, 112
Veggie Sushi, 143
squash, yellow, in Ancient Millet Harvest, 149
Standard Smoothie, 57
Steak, One Great, 140
Steak Fries, 124
Steak Salad, Exotic, 118
stews. *See* soups and stews
strawberries
Punch It Up, 60
Smooth Smoothie, 73
Standard Smoothie, 57
Strawberry Spinach Salad, 115
Super Deluxe Smoothie, 69
Sugar Meringues, 169
Sunshine Salad, 114
Super Deluxe Smoothie, 57
Sushi, Veggie, 143
sweet potatoes, in Roasted Roots, 123
sweet potatoes, in Steak Fries, 124
Sweet Rice Vinaigrette, 177
sweets. *See* desserts
Sweet Shake, 59
Swordfish, Baked, 148

tahini, in Halvah, 170
Tahini Dressing, 180
Tamales, 156–157
tapioca flour
about, 26
Cinnamon Rolls, 50–51
Pizza Dough, 88–89
Puff Rolls, 84–85
Rosemary Focaccia, 90–91
Wheatish Bread, 92

teas, 25
Tea Tonic, Green, 70
teff flour
about, 26
Lace Crepes, 82
Seafood Gumbo, 104–105
Tepoz Salad, 112
Teriyaki Marinade, 175
tofu, in Miso Soup, 107
Tofu Cauli Curry, 155
tomatoes
Gazpacho, 109
Mushroom Tomato Soup, 106
Nightshade Sauté, 152
Tropical Twist Smoothie, 58
Truffles, 165
turnip, in Roasted Roots, 123

V-8000, 63
vegetables. *See also specific vegetables*
Chicken Vegetable Soup, 95
Purely Vegetable Soup, 102
Steamed Veggies, 121
V-8000, 63
Veggie Sushi, 143
vinaigrettes. *See* salad dressings
vinegars, 24

walnuts
Buckwheat Banana Bread, 79
Cinnamon Rolls, 50–51
Pumpkin Bread, 81
watermelon, in Summertime Salad, 117
Wheatish Bread, 92
Wild Rice, 130

xanthan gum, 26

yams, for Steak Fries, 124
yogurt, in Standard Smoothie, 57

zucchini, in Ancient Millet Harvest, 149
Zucchini Pasta, 145